MIND & BODY
Metamorphosis

**Conditioning Techniques For
Personal Transformation**

DR MATTHEW MILLS

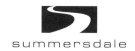
summersdale

Published by Summersdale Publishers Ltd.

46 West Street, Chichester, West Sussex

PO19 1RP United Kingdom

www.summersdale.com

ISBN 978-1-84024-549-3

IMPORTANT NOTE

If you believe you may have a medical condition, the techniques outlined in this book should not be attempted without first consulting your doctor.

Some of the techniques in this book require a high level of fitness and suppleness and should not be attempted by anyone lacking such fitness.

The author and the publishers cannot accept any responsibility for any proceedings brought or instituted against any person or body as a result of the use or misuse of any techniques described in this book or any loss, injury or damage caused thereby.

With thanks...

I would like to thank all those who have supported me in the completion of this volume. I am especially grateful to Alan Gibson for his efforts as editor. Thanks to Clive Kent for his superb design work. I am obliged to Nicky Douglas of Summersdale for her support and guidance in bringing this volume to market and Dr Jennifer Morris for her patience in proofreading.

There are others, too numerous to mention, friends present and absent, for whose contribution to my life I remain eternally indebted. If our character is known from the company we keep, I am truly blessed.

About the Author

Matthew Mills obtained an honours degree in Physiology from the University of Leeds in 1989. He achieved his Masters degree in Human and Applied Physiology from King's College in 1990. Matthew was awarded his PhD from the Department of Medicine, University College London, in 1994. He went on to lecture in Sports Physiology and Health Promotion at the University of Birmingham, Department of Sport and Exercise.

In 1997 Matthew founded The Radical Health Strategy Group, drawing together diverse interests in workplace health promotion from the public and private sector. He led the group's contribution to the Government Green Paper, Our Healthier Nation, in 1998. He remains active in the field, contributing to the Department of Works and Pensions and Health & Safety Executive Stress at Work initiative. Matthew is widely published on the subject of stress in the workplace and is a regular conference speaker. Matthew consults for the Leadership and Cultural Change consultants, Capstone International and ZOOM, whose clients have included British American Formula One Racing, Reuters, Johnson & Johnson, Pro-drive Rally and VISA. He has designed stress management and executive training packages for all of these clients. Matthew is also Director of MK Wealth Management, a City-based IFA and investment broker.

Matthew has studied martial arts for nearly 20 years. He took up karate at the age of 18, expanding his interest to study Eastern culture and Buddhism. Matthew took up kung fu during travels to Hong Kong and China, and has studied Wing Chun under the likes of Yip Chun, whose father taught Bruce Lee. He has developed executive training packages based on these studies, aimed at enhancing fitness, health and mental focus, delivered through Performance First.

Matthew is 38, father to one son – Ben – and lives in London.

Contents

Foreword I

Congratulations on purchasing this book. When Matthew first came to me with his idea for this manuscript, my first reaction was, 'Why didn't I think of that?' You see, I write martial arts books myself and have maintained a reasonable physique into middle age almost entirely by performing related exercises.

However, after getting over my initial irritation, I found Matthew to be not only a very easy person to work with but also very knowledgeable and eminently qualified to talk on the subject. Also, although Matthew's seminars in this field are highly sought after, he is not someone who merely talks the talk – he also walks the walk. His shape, evident on the front cover, bears witness to the success of this method.

The most significant thing I found different in this system – when compared to others – was the fact that Matthew consistently considers and addresses the everyday psychological issues that are bound to rear up at some point. This concern is something that most diet or exercise systems completely neglect and, in my opinion, this (along with the fact that they tend to be boring) is why they almost always fail. The other difference, of course, is that this book is the only equipment you will need.

Mind and body metamorphosis is a complete and robust exercise system that can be trained anywhere and by anyone. In short, and this is no idle boast, by applying the information available in this book it is entirely possible for you to redefine your mind-set, body and lifestyle. You may find later, that you want to progress further into the functional side of martial arts, or you may just be content to be the proud owner of a fitter, healthier and re-sculpted body. Either way, the only missing ingredient is you. So, remember that martial arts are a journey and not a destination, take the time to read and train thoroughly and enjoy the benefits of a new fighting fitness.

Alan Gibson

Foreword II

Dr Matthew Mills has dedicated his life to mastery; mental, physical and emotional, and this book, *Mind and Body Metamorphosis*, sums up step by step how you can achieve this through the medium of Chi Kung.

I first met Matt at Heathrow airport where we were both about to fly out to Valencia to work with the BAR Honda team on a pre-season team 'tune up', just prior to their best ever F1 season to date. One of the first things I asked Matt was what he did, to which he answered enigmatically, 'Lots of things!' The definition of an enigma in the Oxford English Dictionary is 'a mysterious or puzzling person or thing'. This is an almost perfect description of a man whose identity includes Chi Kung practitioner, athlete, artist, doctor, counsellor, coach and director of his own very successful financial services company.

Now, six years later, I am very proud to call Matt a dear friend. His insight, authenticity, values and 'giant cranium' make him my favourite choice for fascinating dinner conversation and insightful counsel. I have significantly benefited from my friendship with Matt and wholeheartedly endorse this book.

Matt's approach takes principles that have stood the test of time over millennia and transforms them into a practical step-by-step guide which can be applied by anyone. This book is powerful, practical and could transform your mental, emotional and physical well-being.

Barry Holmes, Director, Zoom GB Ltd

Introduction

Mind and body metamorphosis

Life is like a card game;
there's the hand you're dealt,
and there's how you choose to play it

Nehru

Introduction - Mind and body metamorphosis

Not for the first time that day I lay, in not inconsiderable pain, on the stone floor of the training hall. For the past 20 years or so I had been interested in martial arts and 'all things eastern'. In that time I had picked up a great many useful techniques and exercises which I can apply in facing the challenges of daily life. The inscrutable smile of my oriental training partner's face, framed by the sky at which I was looking, told me I still had much to learn…

This book is a distillation of the techniques that I have gathered over two decades' experience within martial arts and eastern philosophies. I have employed this system to help senior managers and executives enhance their performance and improve their readiness to meet the challenges of daily life. To successfully meet the needs of this group, the system needed to deliver techniques which can be learned quickly, applied anywhere and still produce profound results for busy people. Whether you need to keep calm in the face of chaos or simply keep your waistline under control on the road, this system is no nonsense and it works.

The roots of mind and body metamorphosis

Chinese boxing, or kung fu, was first developed by the Shaolin Monks of Northern China as a means to defend themselves from bandits while travelling across the country. The techniques at the root of kung fu were in fact introduced to the monks by Buddha when he arrived in China from India. Buddha found the monks to be in such poor condition that he developed a series of breathing exercises for them to practise. Over hundreds of years, these breathing, meditation, boxing and callisthenic exercises evolved into a highly efficient, scientific training system, putting mind and body in a state of readiness for confrontation.

Eastern wisdom for the western world

Consistent with its roots, kung fu does not in fact mean martial art, boxing or even fighting. The term kung fu, which does not have a simple translation into English, really means attainment. Developing fighting ability, or martial kung, is only one element of kung fu. Attainment can also be expressed as learning to remain calm under trying circumstances, to maintain physical constitution against the effects of age or inactivity, or simply improving ourselves through better knowledge of our own abilities. Fortunately, life and death fights are rare these days for most of us. However, these other areas of attainment make kung fu as relevant as ever today – maybe even more so.

Eastern strategies for fitness

The last decade or so has seen an explosion of fitness training as a means to better physical condition and health. Therefore, it is fair to ask whether mind and body metamorphosis will help you become fit. An even more important question is just what we mean by fitness.

Fitness is a fairly vague term, usually taken to mean something like being lean, muscular and able to run a mile or two without too much trouble. Fitness for one person, however, may mean little to someone else. A long-distance runner is fit if they can endure for miles at a time, but they would probably not be fit to enter a weightlifting competition as their training is not geared to the demands of lifting heavy weights. Fitness is more properly defined by the demands of what we are doing and our readiness to meet them.

Demands of daily life

Whether you are a specialist in a particular sport or not, we all share the demands of daily life. The last hundred years in particular have seen an unprecedented transition in the way we live. We have moved from a rural economy, in which most of us performed manual work, toward largely sedentary occupations, in which the principal burden is the accelerating pace of technological change. As a direct result, we are becoming increasingly anxious and depressed, overweight and under muscled, prematurely aged and vulnerable to disease.

Mind and body metamorphosis for everyday readiness

Everyday readiness, and the training to attain it, are defined by the demands of our lives. The following list could doubtless be expanded, but evidence suggests our readiness attainment strategy should target:

Self-confidence - maintaining a positive view of ourselves.
Weight control - maintaining body fat at reasonable levels.
Age prevention - maintaining the strength of muscle and bone.
Disease prevention - maintaining the health of internal organs such as the heart.

Mind and Body Metamorphosis delivers these objectives with a training syllabus systematically directed towards:

Mental relaxation - the ability to enjoy life and see things calmly.
Breathing and mobility - the ability to move joints freely and breathe fully.
Stamina - the ability to keep going and have energy to spare.
Strength - the ability to carry and lift with ease.

The logic of such a syllabus or routine should be self-evident, and there are various exercise systems based on it. A typical exercise programme will, however, usually fail to deliver on its promise. This is not necessarily the fault of the strategy itself, but rather the participant's inability to keep interested and involved. The effects of exercise are short-lived, lasting hours or days, and only continued participation will deliver lasting results. Most fitness and health promotion programmes retain only 5–10% of entrants, so few enjoy much benefit. In addition to the basic elements of a readiness attainment, the strategy must itself deliver the key elements which evidence suggests will keep us interested. In addition to its basic objectives, the advantages of mind and body metamorphosis are:

Inclusive - anyone can join in.
Confidence - systematically develops a positive attitude.
Challenge - enough difficulty to grow, but not put us off.
Progression - seeing and enjoying improvements.
Variety - enough scope to change the strategy.
Enjoyment - scope to imagine, play and have fun.
Convenience - no special equipment or clothing required.
Portability - can be performed anywhere.
Flexibility - adaptable to time and personal constraints.
Adaptability - applicable to our own objectives.
Range - good for groups or those who would rather exercise alone.

Mind and body metamorphosis and life-long readiness

The exercises are arranged in a rough order of difficulty, in a sequence designed to develop a relaxed mind, positive focus, enhanced stamina and enhanced muscular power. This is not dissimilar to the natural evolution of kung fu itself. Each series of exercises forms the foundation for easy progression to the next. While they at first appear novel, each exercise is thoroughly illustrated with easy-to-follow steps.

The kung fu system implicitly includes elements to help us remain encouraged and keep practising over the long term. I have included interesting variations for many exercises, along with advanced alternatives and routines for specific objectives. These are all graded by colour (like the belt systems in judo and karate) so you can choose exercises appropriate for your own ability or level of comfort. Almost anyone can therefore engage in these exercises at some level and observe progression.

I have included elements explicitly aimed at breaking down barriers to practice. The system of exercises is sufficiently flexible to adapt to almost any need, location or time constraint, and guidelines have been provided for this. Further, realising the mind's direction is essential to success; there are specific strategies to help preserve your enthusiasm and prevent the urge to give up. The resulting system is direct, complete and effective.

Using this book

This book is grounded in the idea that a strong mind will overcome a strong fighting technique, and a strong technique will overcome a strong body. Each chapter is designed to help you understand your objective, provide the best techniques to reach it, and develop the foundation for further growth. Rather than presenting a series of disjointed exercises for you to blindly follow, the book is essentially a syllabus through which to progress, master and bend to your will. So, use this book to help develop a stronger mind and direct it through technique to create a stronger body.

The mind and body metamorphosis syllabus

Mind and body metamorphosis is delivered over a 12-week period.

Starting out with developing calm focus we progress through increasingly more demanding stages from Yellow to Black. As we master one series of skills, another is added at the most basic level. Each part of the syllabus develops key skills to get the most out of the following stages. We begin with calm focus to put us in the right frame of mind to get the most out of training. Chi Kung breathing gives us a strong foundation for the demands of stamina training. Developing muscular power begins halfway through the course and only when we have properly conditioned ourselves for the demands of hard work through a few weeks of stamina training.

Week	Calm Focus	Chi Kung	Stamina	Muscle power
1	Yellow	Yellow		
2	Red	Red		
3	Blue	Red	Yellow	
4	Black	Blue	Red	
5		Blue	Red	
6		Black	Blue	
7			Blue	Yellow
8			Blue	Red
9			Black	Red
10				Blue
11				Blue
12	Black	Black	Black	Black

The martial arts from which this book evolved are more than systems for fighting; at their deepest level they are systems of thought and a way of life. Mind and body metamorphosis will not teach you to fight, but by the end of the 12-week syllabus it will equip you to face many other important, and hopefully more frequent, challenges in daily life. Ultimately, wherever you go in that journey, these exercises are a tool to help you get the most from it.

Calm focus
Creating the right frame of mind

The mind's direction
is more important than its progress
Mahatma Gandhi

Calm focus 1.0 - Creating the right frame of mind

What is focus?

Some people always seem to get what they want, while others constantly miss the mark. The difference between them is often the ability of successful people to focus the power of their mind on achieving their goals. We can define focus as attention on a specific goal. This idea also has the deeper connotation of directing our thoughts, will and actions to attaining that goal. The study of the mind pre-dates written history; from the first time one human being wondered why another was acting in a given way. Perhaps later this prompted the questioner to ask the same questions of themselves: 'Why am I doing this and how do I feel about it?' The scientific discipline of psychology was born of these questions and is a relative newcomer on the scene, having only been around for a hundred years or so. As such, it is a little short on definitive answers about why we think, act and feel the way we do. There are, however, some common patterns in human behaviour which give us clues as to why some people can successfully reach their goals, and others can't.

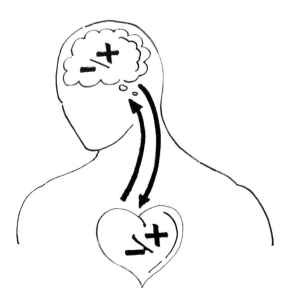

Feel, think and act positively

When you find yourself in the company of focused people it becomes very clear that they know what they want. Whether it's losing weight, succeeding in business or making a relationship work, they can see how to get there and they feel confident that they can do it. When you talk with them, focused people tend to be positive and upbeat. Their enthusiasm is often infectious, it carries them (and those around them) over problems to great achievements. Focused people seem to get lucky, but on closer inspection it becomes clear they make their luck with careful and systematic planning of how they will reach their goals. The benchmarks and milestones of success are clearly laid out, with specific actions and skills practised at each stage to ensure the final outcome. When things go wrong – as they surely will – focused people don't turn the situation into a drama. They view events in a calm, realistic way and then try, positively, to turn things around. Even when they go off the rails and lose focus – and who hasn't – they still see no reason to quit. Lessons can be learnt from failure and focus should return even stronger! In short, focused people have learned a valuable lesson: how you think affects how you feel, how you act and ultimately what you get. Psychology has been successful in giving us a way to systematically improve all of these elements of focus.

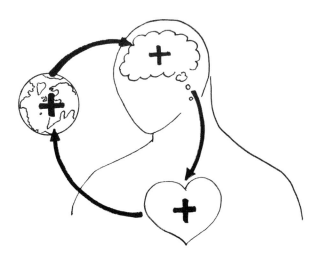

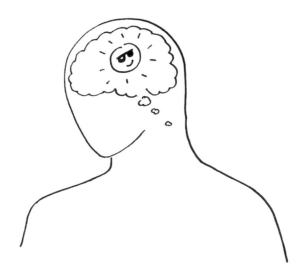

Benefits of learning to focus

Focus exercises can, and should, be performed as often as possible. Developing the habit of positive focus will deliver:

- Less stress, consistently better mood and improved health.

- More energy, enthusiasm and effort toward your goals.

- Better relations with those around you, which may also help you reach your goals.

Guidelines for developing focus

- Practise as often as you can to make positive focus a habit.

- Practise with an open mind.

- Take the time to master each exercise. There is no rush.

• Begin your practice in a quiet, peaceful place.

• Once you have mastered the techniques, practise whenever you can.

• Try and apply your practice to everyday situations and constantly improve yourself.

Using these exercises

Learning to create focus and motivational focus is a complex skill, based on a series of relatively simple building blocks. The following pages lead you through the steps to developing a positive outlook on your goals and also show you how to reach them. Work through each step, being sure to understand it, before proceeding to the next. Leaving any step out weakens the overall effect. Like learning to walk, reshaping our patterns of thinking, which have been ingrained over a lifetime, takes a while – you can expect to fall over a few times. These are among the most difficult skills in this volume, but once mastered you will take the greatest step of all toward realising your goals.

Calm focus 1.1 - Take a deep breath
Level: Yellow

Explanation

We have all had the experience of life getting on top of us. Too much to do and not enough time to do it in. It is very difficult to focus under these conditions and all too easy to lose track of where we are and what we're doing. When it all gets a bit too much, you just have to close your eyes and take a deep breath. This is an in-built reflex which helps us calm down. As we will explore in the following chapter on Chi Kung, deep breathing slows the heart rate, helps us feel more relaxed and focuses the mind. A calm mind is essential to develop focus and for the motivation-building exercises that follow. As you progress through this section, practise the following exercise at the beginning of each session.

Performance

1. Find somewhere quiet where you won't be disturbed.

2. Sit or lay down in a relaxed posture.

3. Close your eyes and take a long, deep breath. Repeat this a few times until you begin to relax.

4. Focus your attention on your legs and feel them relaxing. If it helps you to say or think the word 'relax' – or some other word that works for you – do so.

5. Keeping your eyes closed, slowly shift your focus up your body, feeling all your muscles relax.

6. Take a few more long, slow, deep breaths.

7. Keeping your eyes closed, and continuing to breathe slowly, try to create an image in your mind of somewhere you find pleasant and relaxing. This could be a beach, a wood, a garden – whatever works for you. Try and add some colour to the scene, feeling warm sunshine on your face, smelling flowers – once again, visualise whatever helps you.

8. If you can't imagine a scene, try thinking of a colour you find relaxing – it doesn't really matter, so long as the end result is the same; something that helps you to relax and feel calm.

9. Hang in there for a few minutes, then slowly open your eyes and take another deep breath.

10. Have a bit of a stretch – this feels good too – and then walk around for a minute or so.

Variations

You can practise this sequence almost anywhere. You can be sitting at your desk at work, on the train or anytime at home. Equally, any part of this exercise is useful, from taking a deep breath to imagining a scene that helps you relax.

Benefits

The ability to relax is an amazingly useful and beneficial skill. As we'll see later, a calm mind helps us to think more clearly, making us more focused on our goals and effective in reaching them. Evidence also suggests that relaxation provides us with a range of health benefits, such as lower blood pressure and reducing the chance of heart disease. On a social level, relating to our friends and colleagues is infinitely easier, more pleasant and productive when we are calm and relaxed. Investing a few moments in using these skills clearly provides massive benefits for many areas of our lives.

Calm focus 1.2 - Keep it real

Level: Yellow

Explanation

The way we feel has a profound influence on how we think and act. For example, if you've had a bad day, you may well end up feeling low, you might begin thinking the world is against you and collapse on the couch for a fairly unproductive night of TV. So, when we feel down we tend to think in an unrealistically negative way and our behaviour may follow the same pattern. Fortunately, this process can be put into reverse. If we can think positively, we will feel better and be more likely to act positively. This will help us to stay focused on our goals and we'll be less likely to get side-tracked by problems. The skill of positive thinking – keeping it real – is a powerful tool which can be picked up quickly and, once learned, it soon becomes a habit.

Performance

1. Grab a pen. Using the notes section at the back of this book write down something that happened that made you feel low.

2. Write down some words to describe how you felt, e.g. upset, low, frustrated, angry…

3. Write down what you were thinking when you felt this way, e.g. 'I've failed', 'I should be able to do this', 'how dare they do this to me!'…

4. Now have a good look at what you were thinking. Our thinking often becomes unrealistically negative when we're down or upset.

5. Write down what you ended up doing when you thought this way e.g. 'couldn't be bothered', 'had an argument about it'…

6. When we feel negative, our actions that follow are often unproductive.

7. Now write down what a good friend (someone who knows you, likes you and is sympathetic to you) would say to you to help you feel better, if the same thing happened again.

8. The statement from a friend is likely to be more realistic, positive and sympathetic to us. Hearing this statement makes us feel better.

9. Write down a few more examples of situations which have caused you to feel negative.

10. Write down what you were thinking and then what a friend would say.

11. Every time a situation emerges which makes you feel down, go through this process. Be sure to write things down at first as this helps to ingrain the skill. After a few weeks of practice, it will come naturally.

Example:

- What happened: I put on a few pounds.

- How did I feel: Guilty, frustrated, irritated.

- What did I think: What a failure, I'm turning into a fat slob!

- What did I do: Forget exercise today. Watch TV instead.

- What would a friend say: OK, so you put on a few pounds. That doesn't make you a failure, it happens. Work out and watch your diet for a while and you'll lose it. I know you can do it.

What a friend might say is both more positive AND realistic – it keeps it real.

What a friend might say makes me feel better and more likely to take productive action.

Variations

If you have a friend who will work through some examples with you, that really helps as you'll be getting actual feedback from them.

Benefits

Attitude is everything. If you can stay positive and keep it real you take a giant leap towards reaching whatever goal you set your mind to. Equally, most of us would rather feel positive and happy than down and negative. Changing the way you think can therefore radically improve the quality of your life.

Calm focus 1.3 - Deal with doubt
Level: Red

Explanation

No matter how positively you see the world, every now and again a negative thought appears to undermine even the most upbeat frame of mind. All of us carry demons of one sort or another. Most people spend a fair amount of time grappling with fears, doubts, worries and anxieties. They appear most often when we are down and argue against our thinking positively. Sometime, the more you argue against fears and doubts, the stronger they seem to become. The stronger the demons become, the less likely you are to stay committed to reaching your goals. These demons are known as 'automatic negative thoughts'. While they can seriously undermine your thinking positively and keeping it real, you can readily free yourself of them if you know how.

Performance

1. Go back to the previous exercise, 'Keeping it real'. Read through the example and your own responses again.

2. Focus on the positive and realistic statement a friend may give you when your are down or have lost focus.

3. Think back to a time when this has happened to you. Often we will argue with someone who is trying to make us feel better. These are automatic negative thoughts and they come from fears and doubts we carry with us.

4. In the example below, automatic negative thoughts have been included. Try and think of a time you may have thought like this and how it made you feel.

5. When you practise keeping it real, doubts will crop up. Usually they will follow an attempt to think in a more positive way. e.g. 'I can be successful… but what if I fail…'

6. The best way to deal with these fears and doubts is to accept them. This takes away their power and leaves us able to feel positive.

7. Simply add a statement accepting fears and doubts and they'll soon disappear, e.g. 'I can be successful… but what if I fail…' and so, 'I am bothered by the idea of failing, but everybody is and I'm no different. I will try my best regardless.'

Example:

- What happened: I put on a few pounds.

- How did I feel: Guilty, frustrated, irritated.

- What did I think: What a failure I'm turning into a fat slob!

- What did I do: Forget exercise today. Watch TV instead.

- What would a friend say: OK, so you put on a few pounds. That doesn't make you a failure, it happens. Work out and watch your diet for a while and you'll lose it. I know you can do it.

- Doubt: Yes, but I've tried already and it just isn't working.

- Accept it: I'm afraid it won't work, but sitting on the couch not exercising won't help.

Accepting the doubt not only renders it ineffective, it actually makes keeping it real more powerful.

Variations

Once again, working through some examples with a friend is very powerful. The more often you practise, the better you become at it.

Benefits

Fears and doubts are creations of your own mind. While they do not exist in any real sense, they can have a definite impact on our lives and what we achieve. Many of us will not reach our full potential for no other reason than that we believe that we can't. There is no guarantee that you will succeed, but banishing fear and doubt massively improves your chances – if only because you'll try.

Calm focus 1.4 - Capture confidence
Level: Red

Explanation

Broadly speaking there are two important influences on how we think, feel and act - what happens in the world around us, and our responses. Often we may not succeed, despite a positive environment, because we do not believe in ourselves. Equally, it seems almost no obstacle will stop someone who believes 'I can!' The ideas we have about ourselves – what we should do and how we should be – are often not even our own. We may accept ideas about ourselves which are totally unrealistic – like how we should look and dress – because everyone else seems to buy into them. If we can't live up to these ideas we become negative and disappointed. In the same way as changing the way we think about events can make us feel better about them, we can also change the way we think about ourselves to our advantage. The trick is to create a self-image which is not only positive, but invulnerable to the winds of change or fickle opinions of others. While the world around us may never be certain, our self-belief can become an unshakeable positive force.

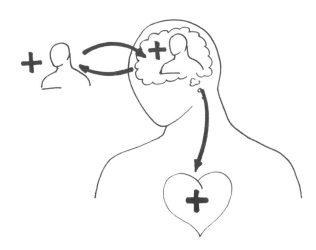

Performance

1. Think how a good friend would describe you and write this down in a few sentences.

2. Now break down the statement into the separate qualities that make you feel good about yourself, e.g. 'I feel good about me because… I'm a nice, generous guy… I always try my best.'

3. Split the qualities up into two groups: those which require you to achieve something for them to be justified and those you'd have regardless of the outcome. For example, you have to do something to justify 'I am successful at work'. You 'try your best' regardless.

4. Write a sentence about yourself based on the qualities in the first group. You are vulnerable where these are concerned because something out of your control may leave you unable to live up to them. For example, it may be important to you to be successful at work, but if someone lets you down you can't finish a job. Not your fault, but you'll feel bad.

5. Now write a sentence about yourself as if a good friend were describing you based only on the items you satisfy regardless of what you do. For example, if you feel good about yourself because you try your best, you'll be positive whatever the outcome of your effort.

6. Focusing on this last sentence you now have an unconditional, positive statement about yourself which you can believe in and feel good about no matter what happens. No one's opinion can change this, and the only measure you have to live up to is your own.

Example:

Ideas about self-image that are conditional and may not be met:

I must be successful

I must look good

I must never fail

Alternative ideas about self-image which are unconditional and can be met easily:

I try my best

I am unique

I accept I'm not perfect

Variations

You can break the idea of positive self-image down into the different areas of your life. You may find it easier to think of self-image in terms of work, family and leisure pursuits.

Benefits

Thinking of ourselves in a positive way is one of the most powerful means to feeling consistently upbeat. To make this work, avoid setting yourself up with ideas which may fail to deliver. Building a realistic view of ourselves, which is positive and can be met whatever happens, is guaranteed to hit the mark. Previously negative situations will have less impact on us, while enhanced self-belief readily translates from improved motivation into higher achievements.

Calm focus 1.5 - See success
Level: Blue

Explanation

Many goals in life can at first seem unattainable. If the very idea of what we're trying to achieve isn't enough to put us off, painfully slow progress toward our objective can lead to our giving up. The key to staying positive and interested in our goals, is to break them down into smaller, more easily achievable steps. Successfully completing each step builds the 'I can do it' feeling, increasing commitment to the next step. This process relies on being realistic about what you want, what you will have to do to achieve it and how long it is likely to take. Systematic planning will soon make success a habit.

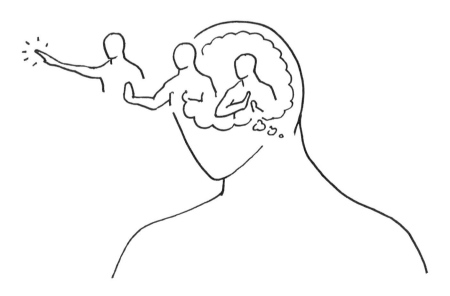

Performance

1. Think about a goal you want to achieve. This could be anything from losing a few pounds or running a marathon, to reaching a business objective or improving a relationship.

2. Write the ultimate goal down – this makes it concrete and real. You'll be amazed how much writing your goal down makes a difference.

3. Think about what progress you could realistically make over the course of a month. If you wanted to lose weight, your monthly goal could be losing 5lbs.

4. Write down weekly benchmarks toward this goal. Using the same example, you would target losing one and a quarter pounds a week.

5. Now write down what you'd have to do, on a week-by-week basis, in order to hit your benchmark. In this example, you'd have to cut a few calories out of your diet each day and exercise vigorously a few times a week.

6. Then consider what you'd have to do on a daily basis to achieve each weekly benchmark. Once again, in this example you'd select low fat foods, eat plenty of fresh fruit and vegetables and program a run or other activity into every other day.

7. Go through this process with your own goals and produce your own benchmarks.

8. Use your benchmarks to show gaps in your knowledge. If you're not sure exactly how to achieve each benchmark, find out more about what you're doing. In the example above you'd find out how many calories are in a pound and a quarter of fat. This would tell you how much you have to cut back on your food consumption each week.

9. You can also use this system to show you how to recover if you go off the rails. If you lapse from your daily or weekly plan, you will know

how far behind your benchmarks you can expect to be. You'll be able to take a realistic view of whether you can catch up or if you have to adjust your benchmarks. Pretty soon you'll be back on track, making progress and putting the lapse behind you.

10. Stick to your daily plan and review your progress against your benchmarks every week. If your progress is not as expected, the fact that you've been systematic means you can easily feed that experience into next week's plan and improve your results.

Variations

You can take this process to almost any level you want. If it suits you to plan down to the last detail, you can. Equally, so long as you stick to the broad principles, you don't have to be obsessive to get what you want.

Benefits

Seeing success on a regular basis is a great way to keep you focused on your goals. Each benchmark you reach rewards you for the effort you have put in. Taking a systematic approach to your goals improves your chances of reaching them immensely. At every step you'll know what to do, why you're doing it and how it will help you get to where you want to be.

Calm focus 1.6 - Feel success
Level: Black

Explanation

An important element of self-belief is being able to visualise ourselves accomplishing our goals. When we can conceive ourselves as being successful, we increase our chances of fulfilling that vision. Visualisation serves as a rehearsal for the real thing. Thinking through the performance of a particular skill trains those parts of the brain associated with movement, programming in better coordination. When it comes to the real thing our performance will be better. The same applies to preparing for specific situations, where we can enhance our readiness by imagining what it would actually be like to be there. Having already experienced the situation in our mind, and considered how we might react, we will deal with it more effectively.

Performance

1. Find somewhere quiet where you won't be disturbed. Close your eyes, take a few deep breaths and relax. Clear your mind of negative thoughts, using the positive thinking skills learned in the previous section 'Keep it real'.

2. Focus your mind on your goal, whatever it may be. Try to imagine yourself when you have reached it. Create an image of where you will be, what it will look like and how you will feel. Add as much colour as possible by imagining who will be there, what they will say to you, what other benchmarks of success you will see, feel, smell and touch.

3. Now focus on an important skill you require to reach your goal. This may be a form of exercise, a work task or other activity.

4. In your mind, run through performing that task perfectly. Imagine what a perfect outcome looks and feels like.

5. Think through the task again, in slow motion. Try to feel every movement or gesture as if it were actually happening.

6. Repeat this process for a few minutes, focusing on every aspect of a perfect performance. If one aspect of a movement or task draws your attention, so much the better – focus there.

7. Focus again on how it will look and feel to succeed in your goal. Create the link between the perfect performance you have seen and your final success.

8. Take a few deep breaths and open your eyes.

9. Repeat this exercise whenever you can and especially before you perform that important skill for reaching your goal.

Variations

To begin with you may find it easier to imagine watching yourself perform a skill or activity. Just like watching TV, most of us are used to watching others in this way. Persevere with trying to imagine yourself performing perfectly, and the result will be far better.

Benefits

Visualisation is a very powerful tool. Physical performance in many activities has been shown to improve through practice of this alone. Equally, seeing yourself successfully reaching your goals becomes a self-fulfilling prophecy. If you can seriously imagine yourself succeeding, you will.

Chi Kung

Developing a strong foundation

A life is not so much measured by the number of breaths,
but the number of moments that take our breath away

Anon

Chi Kung 1.0 - Developing a strong foundation

What is Chi Kung?

Literally, Chi Kung means the art or attainment of energy. The practice of Chi Kung is older than recorded history, and was probably developed in India before being brought to China around 50 A.D. Classical teaching has it that Chi (energy) circulates through the body, moving through pathways called meridians, and that this enables every function of life. Chi (which can also be translated as 'air'), is believed to be collected from our surroundings by the use of specially developed exercises. These exercises focus on breathing using the abdominal muscles. It is supposed that mental focus allows a practitioner to direct Chi to any desired point in their body, to heal illness or give protection from injury. The practice of Chi Kung, has been used ever since, to increase energy, improve physical health and promote mental well-being.

Energy and relaxation through Chi Kung

The jury is still out on the question of Chi, although the obvious health benefits to practitioners are clear. The value of abdominal breathing (and in Chi Kung teaching us to do it), is in no doubt. We know that oxygen, in the air we breath, fuels every activity of our lives. By the same token, your ability to fill your lungs with air affects everything you do. The lungs are inflated by expanding the rib cage and pushing the diaphragm (a sheet of muscle which separates your chest and tummy) down into the abdomen. The lungs are most effectively ventilated only when the diaphragm is used. Abdominal – Chi Kung – breathing allows you to take bigger breaths and bring more oxygen on board. On a higher level, slow, deep breathing has been shown to have important effects on our heart and mental state. Breathing down into the abdomen impacts the flow of blood back to the heart, promoting a reduction in heart rate. This, in turn, is fed back to the emotional centres of the brain to promote a sense of calm and relaxation, with a reciprocal reduction in blood pressure. These effects are virtually the opposite of the symptoms of mental anxiety. Chi Kung allows you to regulate one of the most rapidly spreading epidemics of western society, namely stress and anxiety. Finally, Chi Kung exercises gently stretch, mobilise and strengthen muscles and joints. It is therefore an ideal introduction to exercise, and will also prepare the body for more demanding activity.

Benefits of Chi Kung

Chi Kung exercises can be performed almost anywhere and will provide several key benefits:

- You will develop a greater sense of calm.

- The strength and mobility of muscles and joints will improve.

- This will have a positive impact on your blood pressure, heart and overall health.

- You will perform almost any physical activity to a higher level without becoming breathless.

Guidelines for Chi Kung training

• Keep an open mind. These exercises may seem unusual, but they work!

• Before beginning Chi Kung, clear your mind of all thoughts, especially negative ones.

• Take the time to master each exercise. There is no rush.

• The best time to practise is at the beginning or end of the day.

• Practise outside or in a clean air environment.

• Do not practise when you're in a hurry or cannot give it your full attention.

Using these exercises

These Chi Kung exercises are the most fundamental, and potentially the most valuable, of this volume. Their practice forms the foundation of everything that follows and it is recommend that you work on them for at least a few weeks before moving on – you'll be glad you did! Each exercise forms the cornerstone of the next. While you may eventually discard some of the more basic steps as you advance, make sure you have mastered them first.

Chi Kung 1.1 - Abdominal breathing
Level: Yellow

Explanation

Oxygen fuels every activity of life. We exchange oxygen with the air through our lungs. The more fully we can inflate the lungs, the more efficiently we can get oxygen into our blood and then on to the tissues of our body. There are two principle elements to inflating the lungs: expanding the rib cage and chest, and pushing the diaphragm into the abdomen (tummy). To inflate the lungs fully we must use the diaphragm. As we do, the abdomen will expand. Similarly, to breathe out fully, we must contract the abdomen. This simple Chi Kung exercise helps us learn to do so.

Performance

1. Stand in a relaxed posture, feet shoulder-width apart.

2. Try to clear your mind or think about something positive.

3. Place the palm of your left hand on your tummy, about 5 cm below your navel. Place your right hand over your left.

4. Slowly breathe in, concentrating on breathing down into your abdomen. You'll feel your hands move outward slightly as you do. Be careful not to 'force' the process and don't actively try to push your tummy out, let the breathing do this.

5. When you've inhaled as far as you can, hold for 2 seconds.

6. Now begin to breathe out gently, and press gently with the palms of your hands. Keep going until you reach the end of the breath.

7. Hold for a second or two, release the pressure from your palms and begin breathing in. Do not maintain the pressure with your palms as you breathe in.

8. Continue for 9–10 breaths, then relax your arms to your side and breathe normally.

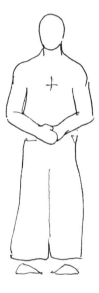

Variations

You can practise this exercise with you eyes closed if it helps. Focus specifically on the movement of your tummy, felt through the palms of your hands. You may imagine the breath being light or golden as you breathe in, dark or black as you breathe out. Equally, you may imagine a light coming on as you breathe in and going out as you breathe out. These are all techniques to focus and calm the mind, focusing on something positive as you breathe in, so feel free to use whatever works for you.

Benefits

The ability to inflate the lungs properly will translate to easier breathing with almost any activity. As you become proficient, the rate at which you breathe will slow and the depth increase. People often say 'take a deep breath' when you're anxious. You may well notice yourself feeling calmer as a result of your practice.

Chi Kung 1.2 - Lifting the sky
Level: Yellow

Explanation

The movements of our whole body can effect the mechanics of breathing. In recognition of this fact, the Chinese developed a series of Chi Kung exercises using specific movements coordinated with breathing. Ultimately, these were integrated with fighting movements to form Tai Chi. In Lifting the Sky, we learn a means of enhancing the expansion of the chest and abdomen (therefore lungs) by coordinating breathing in with a simple arm movement.

Performance

1. Stand in a relaxed posture, feet shoulder-width apart.

2. Place the hands in front of your tummy, palms pointing toward the floor, fingers pointing toward those of the opposite hand.

3. Press your tongue against your palate and breathe through your nose.

4. Slowly breathe in, concentrating on breathing down into your abdomen. As you do so, lift your arms in an arc in front of your body while keeping them straight. They'll end up over your head, palms facing up.

5. As you reach the end of breathing in, push your hands toward the sky. Then hold for a second or two.

6. Relax and gently breathe out while lowering your hands to your sides.

7. Repeat this movement 9–10 times.

8. On the final repetition remain in the relaxed position, concentrating on abdominal breathing for a further 10 breaths.

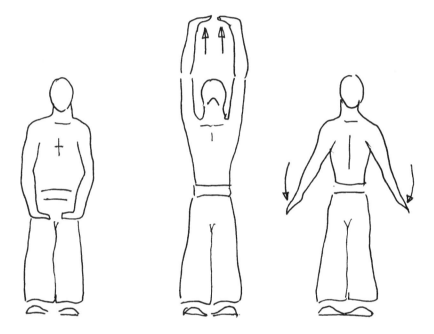

Variations

This movement is fairly proscribed, so to gain the full benefits of practice there aren't really too many variations. The same ideas about having your eyes open or closed apply here, as in the previous exercise.

Benefits

Importantly, this exercise helps us understand how to breathe through movement, which we'll use in later stamina and power training exercises.

Chi Kung 1.3 - Catching the Moon
Level: Red

Explanation

The word 'Chi' is synonymous with 'air' or 'energy' and the translation can almost be used interchangeably. Chinese medicine contends that we draw energy into our body through the air we breath and that this flows through the body along special channels called meridians. The uninterrupted flow of Chi throughout the body is essential to good health and this is the aim of Chi Kung. Catching the Moon introduces a more advanced form of abdominal breathing, reinforced by the movement of the whole body, plus a visualisation technique to help the flow of Chi. Whether you subscribe to the idea of Chi or not, the visualisation technique offers a useful means to focus the mind and coordinate your breathing with movement. Chinese medicine also maintains that a healthy back is central to health and longevity. This fact is self-evident as a weak back will limit or prevent almost any activity. Catching the Moon mobilises the spine and the muscles that support it. Continued practice of this movement will also maintain a healthy back.

Performance

1. Stand in a relaxed posture, feet shoulder-width apart.

2. Place the hands in front of your tummy, palms pointing toward the floor.

3. Using the thumb and forefingers, form an 'O' shape between both hands.

4. Press your tongue against your palate and breathe through your nose.

5. Slowly breathe in, down into your abdomen. Focus your attention through the 'O' between your hands. As you breathe in, lift your arms in an arc in front of your body while keeping them straight. Arch your back and take your hands back over your head, still looking through the 'O' shape, as far as is comfortable. You should end up looking up and back through the gap between your hands. Then hold this position for a second or two.

6. Relax and gently breathe out while lowering your hands to your sides. Continue breathing out and bend forward, reaching with your fingertips toward the ground.

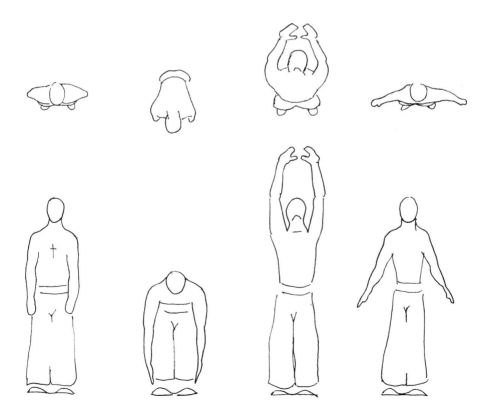

7. When you have fully exhaled, gently breathe in, repeating the whole sequence again.

8. Repeat this sequence a few times, then as you begin to breathe in imagine the air flowing down the inside of your chest into your lower abdomen. As you breathe out, imagine air from your abdomen flowing up your spine and over the back of your head before exiting through your nose. Repeat this sequence a further 7–9 times.

Variations

Visualisation is the key to this exercise. Once you're comfortable with the movement, focus on the flow of air, or Chi, around your body. Different images work for different people, so find one that works for you. Think of the flow of energy as a bright light, stream of water, air, or whatever appeals to you.

Benefits

The coordination of breath, movement and visualisation is central to many martial arts. The ability to achieve this coordination can significantly increase your focus and achievement in almost any physical activity, a fact demonstrated by kung fu practitioners who have mastered this skill. The demands of practising such focus also takes your mind off other concerns, giving you a mental break from day-to-day concerns and promoting mental relaxation.

Chi Kung 1.4 - Three Circle Stance
Level: Red

Explanation

The Three Circle Stance is used extensively in Tai Chi for cultivating the flow of energy throughout the body. The wide stance not only sinks the body's centre of gravity, but is believed to assist the accumulation of Chi in the abdomen. The idea is that this 'reservoir' of energy can then be directed to where it is needed in the body. This may be for the purpose of promoting health, or directing energy through the fists and into an opponent during combat. If you don't like the idea of Chi and energy reservoirs you can think of this as an advanced abdominal breathing exercise. Having mastered the mechanics of abdominal breathing, the real value of this exercise is the deeper level of visualisation, focus and relaxation it promotes. Thus it is a more complete exercise than abdominal breathing alone.

Performance

1. Stand in a relaxed posture, feet about twice shoulder-width apart. Bend your knees and drop your weight about 6 inches.

2. Place the hands in front of your chest, with your hands positioned as if holding a football. Your elbows should be bent and pulled in towards each other just in front of your chest.

3. Slowly breathe in, down into your abdomen. Focus on absolute stillness. At the end of the inhalation, hold your breath for a second or two.

4. Relax and gently breathe out from your abdomen. Throughout, there should be no visible movement of your body, with the exception of your abdomen rising and falling with the breath.

5. Repeat this sequence a few times, then as you begin to breathe in, imagine the air flowing down the inside of your chest into your lower abdomen. As you breathe out, imagine air from your abdomen flowing up your spine, through your shoulders, along your arms and out through your fingers. Repeat this sequence a further 7–9 times.

6. Next, as you breathe in tense the perineal muscle (the ones you clench when you can't find a toilet!). As you breathe in, imagine energy forced to remain in your abdomen, pushed down into your legs and through your feet into the ground. Relax the perinea and breathe out. Repeat 7–9 times. Then, slowly return to a normal standing posture and relax.

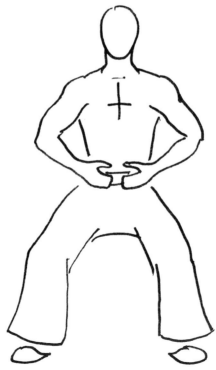

Variations

There are few variations to this exercise as there is little movement. You can practise this posture while holding the lower abdomen as described in the first Chi Kung exercise. Equally, you can use any visualisation technique which works for you. The essential point is to focus on stillness.

Benefits

The wide stance posture provides excellent exercise for the lower limbs as a primer for more demanding physical exercises. The emphasis on physical stillness and singular mental attention will focus and relax the mind. Both qualities will enhance the performance of exercises described later. The focus on stillness is without doubt the most beneficial element of this exercise. Busy lives rarely permit physical or mental relaxation, usually leading to fatigue, anxiety and illness. Learning the skill of being still offers us a degree of protection.

Chi Kung 1.5 - Energy in motion
Level: Blue

Explanation

Just as movement can support proper breathing, as in Catching the Moon, poor coordination can prevent it. Think about a time you have lifted a heavy object, a natural reaction is to tense up and hold your breath. Continued for any length of time, your chest will be heaving as you pant for breath and you'll start running out of energy. From a classical point of view, holding your breath or breathing rapidly prevents a regular intake of Chi, while muscular tension prevents its flow around the body. For those less willing to accept the classical standpoint, we can just as easily use the word 'oxygen' instead of Chi here and the explanation still holds true. If you've ever seen anyone performing Tai Chi and wondered why the movements are so slow and soft, this is the reason. Tai Chi practitioners are developing the flow of Chi within their limbs, in coordination with their breath and movement. The amazing power demonstrated by Tai Chi masters is a testament to the effectiveness of this 'internal' training. So, having learned to breathe with the abdomen, the next advancement in Chi Kung is to regulate your breathing during movement.

Performance

1. Stand in a relaxed posture, feet fairly close. Bend your knees and drop your weight a few inches.

2. Place the hands in front of your chest, palms facing out, fingers pointing upward. You should look like you're just about to push something away from you.

3. Keep your feet where they are and turn your upper body towards your left.

4. Slowly breathe in, down into your abdomen. As you do, lean back slightly and place your weight over your right leg. At the end of the inhalation, hold your breath for a second or two.

5. Relax and gently breathe out from your abdomen. As you start to exhale, slowly step forward with your left foot and push your hands out in front of you. Keep going until your weight is over the left leg, arms extended and you have fully exhaled. Keep your movements slow and graceful. Imagine power rushing from your abdomen, through your shoulders and down through your hands.

6. Keep your feet where they are and slowly breathe in, down into your abdomen. As you do, draw your hands back to your chest and shift your weight back over your right leg. At the end of the inhalation, hold your breath for a second or two.

7. Slowly exhale and push forward again.

8. Repeat up 9 times. At the end of the last movement, keep your arms extended and turn your torso to the right. Now repeat the process on this side.

9. At the end of the next cycle, turn to face forward again and assume the Three Circle Stance for a few breaths. Then slowly assume a normal standing posture and relax.

10. As you advance in Chi Kung you'll find each breath becoming deeper and longer. The next phase is to repeat the movement cycle several times during one breath. After a few weeks of consistent practice you may find yourself able to repeat two pushes forward, at the same speed, for one breathing cycle.

Variations

You can try this kind of breathing with almost any movement. The key is to keep movements slow and relaxed, focusing on your breathing and visualisation.

Benefits

Consistent practice of these exercises will very quickly pay dividends. The ability to coordinate deep breathing, muscle relaxation and mental focus will help improve both your level of energy and resistance to fatigue. Don't be surprised if many activities which used to cut you down to size with aching limbs and gasping breath become less of a challenge.

Chi Kung 1.6 - The Thousand Steps
Level: Black

Explanation

Kung fu masters can spar for hours without becoming tired or breathless. Their secret?; a form of breathing control called the Thousand Steps. This exercise aims to develop a reserve of Chi, or energy, which is always carried in the abdomen to fuel physical exertion. Once again, for those whose focus is more firmly fixed on contemporary science; the typical response to physical exertion is panting, taking shallow breaths using the chest, or not breathing at all. The Thousand Steps teaches us to buck this trend and ensure the lungs are always working to capacity, feeding oxygen to the body. As a word of caution, this is an advanced technique which will prepare you for the stamina and strength exercises later in this volume. Do not attempt this exercise unless you have mastered abdominal breathing and practised regularly.

Performance

1. You'll need to be somewhere open like your garden or local park.

2. Stand in a relaxed posture and clear your mind.

3. Perform abdominal breathing 3 or 4 times.

4. Slowly breathe in, down into your abdomen. At the end of the inhalation, hold your breath for a count of five.

5. Keep your mouth slightly open and allow yourself to slowly exhale. Your breath should escape naturally and without conscious effort.

6. When you feel you have breathed out 70% of a full exhalation, breathe deeply into your abdomen and repeat the cycle. At no point should you reach the point where you feel breathless or distressed. If this happens you are either;

- not ready, and should go back to practising abdominal breathing for a while,
- not inhaling fully using your abdomen,
- or, you are forcing the breath hold for too long and not allowing breath to escape naturally.

7. Next, and only when you're comfortable, start walking. Focus on deep inhalation, holding your breath and allowing 70% to escape naturally before inhaling again. It will take a while to get used to, so start walking only slowly and for short periods. Rest and then go at it again.

8. Gradually, extend the period of breath holding and exhalation. Then pick up the duration and speed of your walking until you can take a thousand steps.

Variations

This breathing technique can be applied to almost any physical activity and will improve your endurance. Hold in mind to start slowly when applying this technique to a new activity, probably about half your normal pace, and build up gradually.

Benefits

The Thousand Steps is a great achievement in your Chi Kung training. The effort you put in, will have an amazing impact on your physical performance and endurance.

Developing stamina
Wing Chun kung fu exercises for endurance and weight control

The longest journey starts with the first step
Lao Tsu

Stamina training 1.0 - Wing Chun kung fu exercises for endurance and weight control

How stamina training works

Whenever we want to lift or move something, we have to produce the force to do so in our muscles. This process requires energy, and the more muscles we use at one time, the more energy we require. The fuel to drive our muscles comes from the food we eat and the oxygen we breathe. Muscles have enough fuel built in for short bursts of work (anaerobic), but to continue for longer periods they must be supplied by additional oxygen resources from the blood, pumped by the heart (aerobic). The more muscles we use, the more energy we require, so the heart must work harder to provide oxygen – as a result we must breathe harder.

Stamina training helps us to increase our readiness to perform longer bouts of work, exercise or play. There are three vital links in this process:

- Breathing properly, to get the maximum amount of air and oxygen into the lungs.

- Training the heart to deliver oxygen rich blood to the muscle.

- Training the muscles to use oxygen more efficiently.

Combined arm and leg stamina training

The best way to train for stamina is to use as many muscles as possible, for prolonged periods. The most effective way to accomplish this is to exercise our arms and legs at the same time. Combined arm and leg exercise produces the greatest overall workload, and therefore training for the heart and breathing. Equally, as many muscles as possible are trained to use more oxygen. This is the basis for kung fu stamina training.

Benefits of stamina training

Stamina training will deliver a number of valuable benefits. Most important are:

• The heart becomes stronger and less prone to disease, especially coronary artery disease.

• The chemistry of the blood changes to further reduce the chance of heart disease, mainly by lowering cholesterol which contributes to coronary artery disease.

• Blood pressure (associated with 50% of all deaths when elevated) tends to lower.

• We become more able to sustain heavy exercise. Previously difficult activities feel easier.

• Our resistance to fatigue goes up, we have more energy and recover more quickly when tired.

• The high levels of energy expenditure (highest during combined arm and leg exercise) helps weight control.

Guidelines for stamina training

There are no hard and fast rules, but here are some pointers for stamina training:

• Don't train for an hour after eating or an hour before doing so.

• Drink plenty of water and keep hydrated.

• Do not exercise if you have drunk alcohol beforehand and refrain from smoking.

• A specific warm-up is probably not required, but start at around 50% of your top effort and build up the effort over a few minutes.

• Work at a level which makes you breathe hard, but where you're not fighting for breath.

• Work continuously and rhythmically in any stamina exercise.

• Throw in bursts of intense effort now and then to really push yourself.

• Train at this pace for 20–30 minutes 4–5 times a week.

• Focus on combined arm and leg exercises, and specifically using large muscle groups, like the shoulder girdle, back and legs.

• Train for stamina before you train for strength, as power training will tire you out.

• Ease down gradually from maximum effort, don't just stop.

Using these exercises

These exercises will systematically develop your stamina. Each exercise builds the foundation for the next. Be sure to work through the exercises in order, progressing to the next level only when you have mastered the previous one. There is no rush and you will not get the most from your training if you neglect the basic foundations. Patience and diligent practice will reward you with far greater and more sustainable results.

Stamina training 1.1 - The character two stance
Level: Yellow

Explanation

The Character Two Stance is named after the Chinese character which the stance resembles. This is the basic training stance of Wing Chun kung fu and the foundation for all the techniques we'll use later. The arms and legs are positioned to protect vital points along the centre line of the body (head, heart and groin) while not committing the body in any particular direction. Like the tennis player awaiting a serve, the Character Two Stance leaves you ready to react and move in any direction.

Performance

1. Stand with your feet together, hands by your sides.

2. Bend your knees slightly, dropping your body about 10 cm.

3. Keeping your heels in place, turn your feet outwards at least 45 degrees.

4. Now keep the balls of your feet in place and turn your heels outward so your feet end up pointing inward about 45 degrees.

5. Push your backside forward, rotate your pelvis upward and press your knees inwards so there is about one fist distance between them. Your legs and buttocks should be tensed.

6. Place your left hand, palm facing in and fingers pointing upward, about 10cm from the centre of your chest.

7. Place your right hand, palm facing in and fingers pointing forward, in front so that the elbow is alongside the left hand. This is your guard. Now you're ready to rumble!

8. Press your tongue against your palate and breathe gently through your nose.

9. To close the stance, jump your feet together, landing on the balls of your feet. Then lower your feet to the ground, place your hands by your sides and relax.

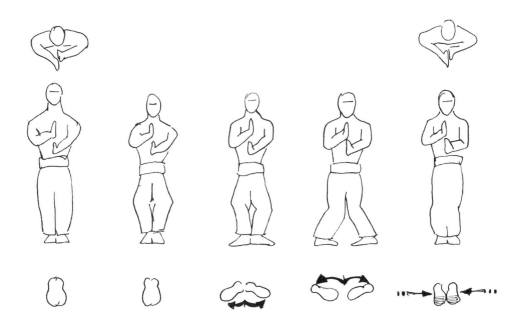

Variations

Practise opening and closing the stances 10 times or more in succession. Practise holding the stance for a minute or more, keeping your legs tensed and breathing steadily as you do. Try performing the Chi Kung exercises in this position. You can also try this stance standing on one leg, pulling the knee toward your chest and holding for as long as you can. When you've mastered this, try standing on one leg, holding the other outstretched in front of you.

Benefits

You'll quickly find that practising this stance tones up your thighs and backside. Climbing stairs will also become easier.

Stamina training 1.2 - Chain punches
Level: Yellow

Explanation

Kung fu contains a huge variety of strikes and punches. The chain punch is used to attack an opponent with a series of repetitive strikes, which are very difficult to defend. The idea is to strike as often as possible. Chain punching utilises muscles from the entire upper body and therefore helps to build stamina in muscle groups that are often neglected. At the same time the waist and legs must also work to provide a stable platform from which to launch the attack. When we consider that 60% of muscle is in the upper body, the potential benefits of this exercise become clear.

Performance

1. Open the Character Two Stance and place your hands in the guard position.

2. Form your hands into a fist with the knuckles aligned vertically and the thumb on top of the hand.

3. With the rear hand, punch down the centre line of the body at nose level. At the same time withdraw the other hand toward the chest under the punch. You'll finish in an on-guard position with hands the other way around.

4. Practise this movement until you can punch smoothly, hand over hand. The movement is not unlike cycling the pedals of a bike with your hands.

5. Practise cycles of 3, 5, 7 and 9 punches non-stop. Try to punch as fast as you can, without losing the form of the punch.

6. Gradually build up the number of punches until you can perform a minute non-stop.

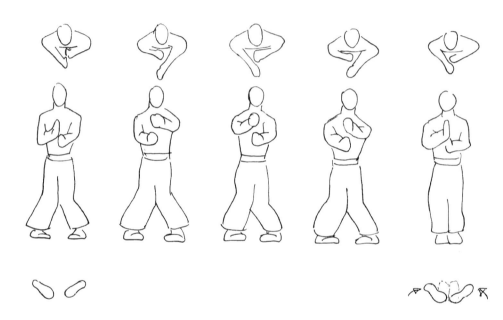

Variations

Practise launching a series of punches at waist height, chest height and head height. Try launching punches off to your left and right-hand side. For added variety try cycling the hands in the reverse direction. The rear hand comes forward, under the lead arm as you pull it back. You may want to open your hand for this variation as you are pushing an opponent away.

Benefits

Few exercises target the upper body for stamina training and fewer still will tax them like chain punching. Results will come quickly in terms of the tone, shape and stamina of the entire upper body.

Stamina training 1.3 - Squat and kick
Level: Yellow

Explanation

The legs are more powerful than the arms and have a longer reach. Kicking, and training the leg muscles forms an important part of kung fu. Different forms of kung fu emphasise different kicking techniques. All have in common the need for strong muscles to execute the kick and, more importantly, to support the body weight on one leg while doing so. The squat and kick exercise is a basic exercise to accomplish this aim.

Performance

1. Open the Character Two Stance and place your hands in the guard position.

2. Squat down, keeping your back straight, until your thighs are parallel with the floor.

3. Push up rapidly, driving the right foot up from the floor and outwards to strike an imaginary opponent on the shin using your heel.

4. Recover the kicking foot to the starting position.

5. Repeat the squat, kicking out with the left foot.

6. Practise 5, 10, 15 and 20 kicks on each side until you can keep going for a whole minute.

7. Speed up the pace of the exercise as you improve.

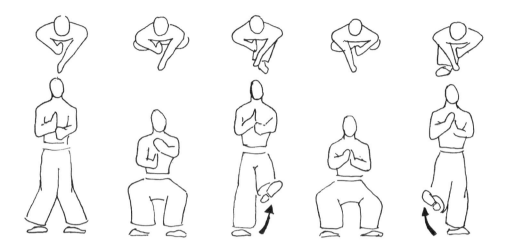

Variations

Practise launching kicks alternately at shin, knee and waist height. As your flexibility improves you may wish to kick higher. You may wish to switch your guard hands around as you kick, i.e., right hand forward as right leg kicks. An added twist is to punch out on the same side as you kick. Add another dimension to the exercise by chain punching after each kick or even throughout the entire exercise.

Benefits

This simple exercise is a fabulous conditioner for all the muscles of the lower body. Your breathing after one minute will attest to the amount of work you are doing and thus conditioning for your heart. Adding chain punches means you will be working over 95% of the muscle in your body and establishing a firm foundation for all the exercises to come.

Stamina training 1.4 - Turning Stance and Asking Hand

Level: Red

Explanation

You may have the most devastating fighting techniques in the world, but if you can't direct them toward your opponent, you're like a cannon without wheels. This exercise shows how to turn the Character Two Stance. The body turns and the guard swings out towards your adversary while you prepare to face them. This arm movement is called Asking Hand. This movement also sets up the kung fu fighting stance from which we'll begin to add a new, dynamic element to our exercise.

Performance

1. Open the Character Two Stance and place your hands in the guard position, right hand forward.

2. Keeping your heels in place, turn the toes of the right foot outward.

3. Now, two things happen at once: swing 90 degrees around to the right from the waist while swinging your right arm out to the right side, so the hand ends up at eye level and palm down. Try to keep your hips roughly in line with your shoulders as you perform this action.

4. Most of your weight should be on your back leg (as a test, you should be able to lift the right leg off the ground while remaining steady on the back, left leg).

5. Once you've swung around to face the right, place your hands back in the guard position.

6. Return to the starting position by turning the toes of the right foot to point inward at 45 degrees again. Keep your hands where they are and turn the body inward from the waist.

7. Change your guard, so the left hand is forward, and repeat on the left side.

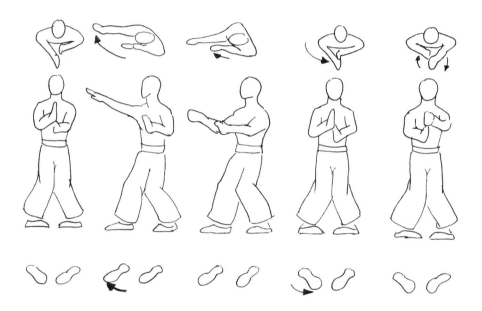

Variations

At the end of the Asking Hand movement, snap your arms forcibly into the on-guard position. Add a series of chain punches before you turn and when you reach the final position of the turn. Imagine you are facing and taking out multiple opponents. You can also throw in a kick at the beginning and end of the turn. Another interesting variation, which will really emphasise those waist muscles, is to turn quickly, left to right, swinging your arms vigorously as you go.

Benefits

Aside from setting up the basic fighting stance, this exercise provides conditioning for the muscles of the waist and shoulder from the swinging arm movement. Pulling together the whole series of movements will also offer an interesting challenge for your coordination.

Stamina training 1.5 - Chain punch and chasing steps

Level: Red

Explanation

Most opponents don't oblige you by standing still when you try to strike them. Particularly against a flurry of attacks, like the chain punch. Most people will try to back away. So, we now have to give chase. This exercise teaches us how to achieve this whilst maintaining the integrity and protection offered by our fighting stance. Chain punching with chasing steps also aids better coordination of the arms and legs.

Performance

1. Open the Character Two Stance and place your hands in the guard position, right hand forward.

2. Using the Turning Stance and Asking Hand, turn to the right and assume the guard position in the fighting stance.

3. Lift the lead leg and step forward.

4. The back foot stays in close contact with the ground and does not move until the lead foot touches the ground. It is essentially dragged up toward the lead to establish the original distance between the feet.

5. Try a few steps with hands in the on-guard position to get the feel of it. When you're ready, throw in a few chain punches as you step.

6. When you reach the wall or boundary of your practice area, or whenever you feel like it, turn using the Asking Hand and go the other way.

7. Practise 5, 10, 15 steps and chain punches in each direction, with turns. When you've got the hang of it, work up to a solid minute of stepping and continuous punching without pause. At this point try to speed up the steps and punches, really going after an imaginary opponent.

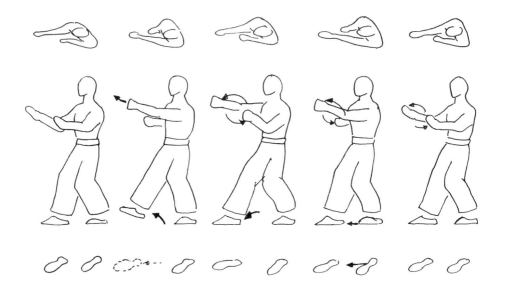

Variations

At the end of a series of steps, try pretending to forcibly push your opponent away from you with both hands, before you assume the on-guard position and turn. You can also try stepping backwards whilst punching. Another variation is to step backward and reverse the hand movement (the rear hand comes up under the forward hand as it is pulled back) and open the hand, as if pushing an opponent away.

Benefits

In addition to working 95% of the muscles in your body, you're also moving the whole body weight around in this exercise. When you move at speed, your energy expenditure here outstrips almost any other exercise. The potential for weight control, and conditioning the heart, are therefore tremendous. Your coordination will improve dramatically with practice and the range of variation lends this exercise to expansion by a playful imagination.

Stamina training 1.6 - Chain punch, kicks and chasing steps

Level: Red

Explanation

This is the next evolution, and natural progression of chain punching and chasing steps. Once we've coordinated the arms and steps in attack and defence, we bring in the big guns with kicking. This exercise adds another layer of coordination and skill, but also takes you up a gear in terms of energy expenditure and conditioning potential.

Performance

1. Open the Character Two Stance and place your hands in the guard position, right hand forward.

2. Using the Turning Stance and Asking Hand, turn to the right and assume the on-guard position in the fighting stance.

3. Before you step, drive the leading foot up from the ground in a kick to an imaginary opponent's shin.

4. Rather than return the kicking foot to its original position, let it fall forward, about the distance of a natural step.

5. Drag the back foot up towards the lead foot, chain punching as you go.

6. Practise 5, 10, 15 or more steps with kicks, punches and turns until you can go for a full minute. Then try and speed up the process, getting in as many moves as possible within a minute.

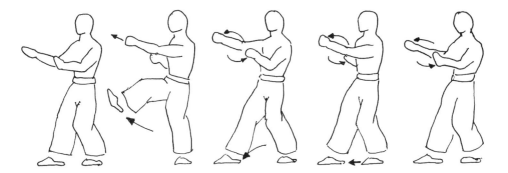

Variations

Try driving kicks to shin, knee, waist level and even higher as your flexibility improves. Try kicking twice before you put your foot down, to the shin, then the waist for instance. When you kick forward, try holding the kicking leg outstretched for a few seconds and chain punching before you set the foot down. Try driving kicks from the back leg, this will change your guard around and the back leg will end up taking the lead position.

Benefits

This exercise offers unsurpassed exercise for the entire body. Even the muscles of the abdomen will be called forcefully into play as you lift your legs to kick. Once you've mastered this technique, and can keep going for extended periods, you will have a tool to promote a level of conditioning which would make most athletes sit up. You are not neglecting a single muscle in your body – and it can all be done in your living room!

Stamina training 1.7 - Boxing rounds, the Rickshaw, side jump and kneeling walk

Level: Blue

Explanation

Having mastered kicking and punching on the move, we're now ready to move on to the next level and add a few more advanced techniques.

Performance

1. Work up your kicking and stepping with chain punches, until you can keep going for a full minute. Now start building a routine by adding a few more rounds of boxing.

2. Work up to 5, one minute rounds, with a minute break between rounds. You can do this simply by adding a round of boxing a day for a week.

3. Gradually extend each round, until you can perform 5 rounds of three minutes When you can do this comfortably, you are now ready to add in some advanced exercises.

4. Lift the knee of the lead leg toward your chest and hop backwards and forwards on the rear foot while chain punching. This is called the Rickshaw. Practise 10, 20, 30 hops on each foot, then continue with steps and punches.

5. Imagine you suddenly see an opponent attacking you from the left side. Jump to the right, landing on the right foot and kicking out at shin level with the left foot. Now look to the right and without putting

the left foot down, jump off the right foot, land on the left and kick out with the right. These are jumping kicks. Practise 5, 7, 10 jumps to each side, keep punching all the time, and then continue with stepping and punching.

6. Keeping the right foot on the floor, kneel on the left knee. Staying as low as possible, step forward so you end up kneeling on the right knee with the left foot on the floor. Practise, 5, 10, 20 steps, punching as you go. Then return to steps and punches.

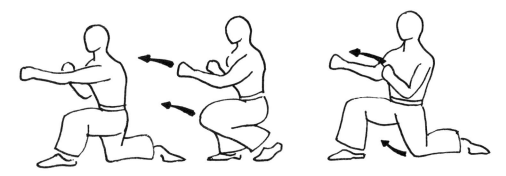

Variations

As you finish a sequence of the kneeling walk, kick out as you stand up. You can also try the Rickshaw with your lifted leg stretched out in front. As you perform the side jump you may want to combine an Asking Hand or punch on the same side as the kick. Throw these exercises into a round of boxing whenever you feel like it. You may also want to drop in a sequence of turns or squat kicking. None are absolutely essential, so if you fall in love with one exercise, feel free to go with the urge.

Benefits

The advanced routine and exercises add a new dimension of workload and variation. The Rickshaw emphasises the muscles of the calf, while the jump kicks and especially the kneeling walk will do things for your thighs and buttocks that you would not believe.

Stamina training 1.8 - Free form
Level: Black

Explanation

The foundations having been thoroughly built, with correct breathing, mental attitude and technique, you're now ready to make up your own form. Free form routines combine all of the skills you have learned, but without rigid structure. The following is a suggested Black level performance and progression, although whether you follow this particular routine is your choice now.

Performance

1. Work up to 10 or more, 3–5 minute rounds, with a 30 second break between rounds.

2. Towards the end of each round consciously push yourself harder, punching faster and kicking more regularly.

3. Throughout the round, throw in bursts of intense effort for 10–20 seconds before returning to your usual pace. Coordinate bursts of chain punches with equally aggressive and rapid chasing steps. Really go after your opponent.

4. Do not limit your self to kicking forward, but try (with caution) kicking in any direction that speaks to you.

5. If you've seen boxing on the television, feel free to incorporate any of the moves you've seen into your routine.

6. Don't just step forward and backward. Step to the side and move around your opponent.

7. Throughout, try to develop your engagement and enjoyment with a little healthy imagination. Imagine you are sparring with opponents coming at you from all directions. If you feel like letting out a 'Wah!' or 'Hiya!' as you strike out, go for it (I'm pretty sure Bruce Lee would approve and it's remarkably liberating!). This will add an element of much needed play to your routine.

Variations

At this stage, while remaining true to the basic techniques which have got you to this point, you should feel free to improvise. An excellent variation, however, which will take you to an even higher level, is the addition of resistance. You may not have any small weights you can hold in your hand while boxing, but canned food serves just as well! They are cheaper and you can pick them up anywhere. Equally, you can apply what you've learned to almost any other stamina exercise. If you like to jog (and you'll have already noticed how your kung fu has improved your running), try holding a tin of canned food in each hand as you run. The weight is small, but the combined effect of arm and leg exercise is impressive.

Benefits

By now you have access to complete conditioning for your whole body, a routine you can perform anywhere with enough scope for growth and variety to maintain your long-term interest. The level of conditioning potential is unrivalled and the possibilities are limited only by your imagination.

Developing power
Wu Shu exercises for developing muscle strength

Anything that doesn't destroy me
makes me stronger

Milo of Crotona

Power training 1.0 - Wu Shu exercises for developing muscle strength

How power training works

Every action of our lives is dependent on muscle. Whether you're performing a complex kung fu move or simply sitting at rest, hundreds of muscles are working together to maintain the position of your limbs. Muscles are composed of thousands of individual fibres. Each fibre is packed with specialised proteins which, when activated by our nerves, cause the fibre to shorten. The shortening muscle fibre pulls on the skeleton and this force causes the joints to move. Muscles become stronger when then are forced to work harder, or produce more force, than normal. Repeated, forceful muscle contractions signal more protein to be incorporated into the muscle, which becomes larger as a result. Larger muscles not only produce more force, but can do more work in a given time, and are said to be more powerful.

Muscle without weight

Most people equate building muscle with lifting weights. In this type of training the muscles are forced to work harder by lifting progressively heavier weights. While there is no doubt that these exercises are effective they require expensive equipment or access to a gym, which may be both inconvenient and unaffordable. An alternative form of power training is to work muscles against themselves, pushing the palm of one hand against the other for instance. Using our muscles to resist our movement is called dynamic tension. We can also position ourselves so that our muscles have to work harder than usual. Standing in a semi-squat for instance, forces the thigh muscle to work harder due to the poor leverage of the muscle around the knee joint in this position. All of these techniques have been developed and refined by Wu Shu (Chinese martial arts) exponents over thousands of years to develop powerful muscles. They are cheap, convenient and highly effective.

Benefits of power training

Training for muscle power is associated with a range of benefits.

• Central among these are:

• Every action of our lives becomes easier, as we have more power at our disposal.

• We are capable of higher levels of physical performance.

• Increased resistance to fatigue from high intensity effort.

• Power training prevents the decline in bone strength and muscle strength with age.

• Power training increases muscle mass and metabolic rate, enhancing the effectiveness of any weight loss regimes.

Guidelines for power training

Interestingly, the widely accepted 'rules' for strength training have little scientific basis. Forceful muscle contractions are essential, but an absolute formula does not exist. Experience will guide you, but based on traditional methods some good pointers are:

• Warm up and finish with some light exercise to prevent strains and enhance recovery.

- Exercise somewhere you can concentrate fully on what you are doing.

- Focus your attention on the muscles you want to exercise.

- Breathe steadily throughout your power training and do not hold your breath.

- Exercise large muscle groups first, like the legs, because this requires more effort.

- Move slowly in each exercise concentrating on maintaining the tension in your muscles.

- Exercise at an intensity which causes your muscle to shake slightly – this means you are getting the most powerful muscle fibres to work hard.

- Push yourself. Muscles only get stronger if they are forced to work to their limit.

- Intense muscular exercise is tough and you should expect it to feel uncomfortable. This said, stop exercising at once if you experience pain.

Using these exercises

These exercises are designed to systematically develop power in all of the major muscles groups. Each level of exercise lays the building blocks for the next, so use them in order. Learning the skills of dynamic tension equips you with a powerful, muscle building tool. Neglecting this skill deprives you of your full potential. Results do take time, but if you work conscientiously and patiently, progress will come.

Power training 1.1 - The Prayer Press
Level: Yellow

Explanation

The Prayer Press introduces power training for the upper body and the concept of dynamic tension. This exercise focuses on the muscles of the arms and shoulder girdle which pull the hands across the chest and push outwards. The idea is to produce tension in one group of muscles by using another group against them. In this case, one arm resists the movement of the other. As one muscle group grows stronger, the resisting group will have to become stronger as well. There are some superficial similarities with isometric exercise here. Rather than holding the limbs static, here we move against and through the tension. This means that we increase strength throughout the entire range of joint motion, rather than in just one position.

Performance

1. Open the Character Two Stance.

2. Place your hands together, as if praying.

3. Point the fingers up and position your hands with thumbs touching the middle of your chest.

4. Now press your hands firmly together and maintain the tension.

5. Breathe deeply and steadily.

6. Keeping the tension on, rotate the hands at the wrist so the fingers point down toward the ground. This should take a second or two.

7. Rotate the hands to point the fingers in front and then push your hands outward as far as possible while keeping the palms tightly pressed together. This should take about 2 seconds.

8. Draw the hands back to the chest and rotate the hands to point the fingers upwards.

9. Start with 5 repetitions and slowly work up to 12 or 15.

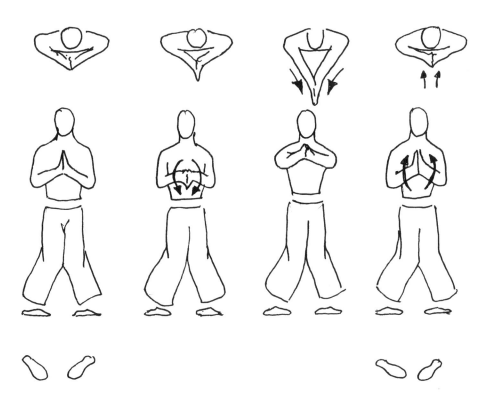

Variations

Try pushing the hands upward or down, rather than just straight out in front. This will emphasise different elements of the shoulder girdle. You could also try pushing the hands out toward the right or left, and this will emphasis one side more than the other. You could also try holding the arms extended for a few seconds – a variation I like is to do this pressing the finger tips together to emphasise the muscles of the forearm. Experiment with holding the extended arm position and describing a large figure eight in front of you.

Benefits

This simple exercise affects almost every muscle of the upper body. Just a few attempts will convince you how hard your muscles are working, and you'll soon find carrying most things becomes noticeably easier. The Prayer Press develops tremendous upper body power and as it can be performed anywhere, it lends itself to further development and experimentation.

Power training 1.2 - The Merry-Go-Round
Level: Yellow

Explanation

The Merry-Go-Round is actually a Shaolin Chi Kung exercise designed to promote the flow of internal energy. Many practitioners report an invigorating effect from this exercise. Whether you subscribe to the idea of 'Chi' touched on in the first section of this book, or not, the Merry-Go-Round provides excellent conditioning for the entire midsection. Most contemporary conditioning programs fall back on sit-ups to firm up the tummy. These exercises neglect the muscles of the back and sides, and also assume a basic level of strength, which may not be available to all of us. The Merry-Go-Round provides a challenge to all of these important muscle groups while the intensity of exercise does not exclude those not yet ready for sit-ups.

Performance

1. Place your feet about twice shoulder-width apart and bend the knees to assume a stable posture.

2. Place your hands together, arms outstretched in front of your chest.

3. Turning from the waist only begin to sweep your arms anti-clockwise in a wide circle.

4. Make a deliberate effort to move through the widest circle possible, leaning as far to the side and backwards as is comfortable for you.

5. Breathe in during the first half of the circle, and out during the second half.

6. Take about 10 seconds for each full circle at first, going in each direction 5 times.

7. Build up to 12–15 circles in each direction. When you reach this number, slow down the rate at which you move until each circle takes 20 seconds.

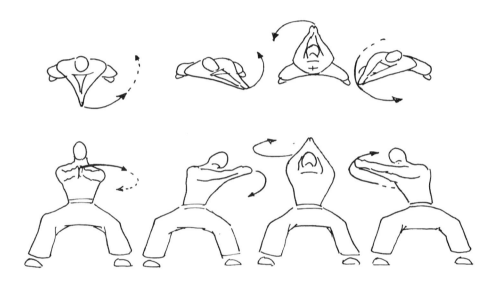

Variations

Some find the hands together uncomfortable, especially when reaching backward at the rear of the circle. You may therefore want to start out keeping you hands on your hips. For the more adept, try stopping and holding your position for 5–10 seconds at each point of the compass as you turn.

Benefits

The midsection forms the lynch-pin about which your body moves. The Merry-Go-Round provides excellent overall conditioning for all muscles of the midsection. Regular practice will help you firm up a soggy tummy without neglecting the strength in the all-important lower back, helping you maintain mobility long into old age. As an added bonus, you may also notice the exercise the thighs get as they work to maintain a stable base for upper body motion.

Power training 1.3 - Horse Stance and Golden Bridge
Level: Yellow

Explanation

Prior to teaching a new student any fighting technique, masters would often insist on a prolonged period of intensive physical training and preparation. The Horse Stance is a fundamental training stance for a huge number of martial arts. It develops power and flexibility in the lower limbs as a strong foundation for other stances. The Chinese also believe that the Horse Stance helps the accumulation of Chi, or energy. The Golden Bridge is a hand form often used in conjunction with the Horse Stance to help to condition the upper limbs, especially the muscles of the forearm which are central to the performance of every hand technique.

Performance

1. Open the Character Two Stance.

2. From the Character Two Stance, perform the same sequence of feet movements again, turning the toes and heels out as before. You'll end with your feet twice shoulder-width apart.

3. Keeping your back straight, sink your bottom down until your thighs are almost parallel with the floor. There is a tendency to lean forward and let the bottom stick out, so concentrate on pushing your pelvis forward and keep the back straight.

4. Once you are comfortable place both hands in front of your chest, palms facing forward and fingers upward.

5. Curl the fingers inward so only your index finger points straight up. Point your thumbs toward each other so the thumbs and index finger forms an 'L-shape'.

6. Breathe in through the nose, then exhale and push your hands out until your arms are straight, keeping the same hand position. If you're doing it right you will feel tension along the top of your forearm.

7. Hold this final position breathing slowing and steadily. Focus on maintaining your hand position and keeping your legs still.

8. Hold this position for 30 seconds to begin with. Work up to a minute by adding 10 seconds every day or so that you practise. Work up to holding the Golden Bridge for 3–5 minutes or so.

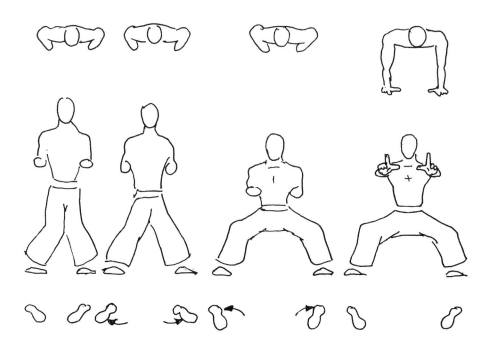

Variations

Instead of holding the arms static, try pulling them in as you inhale and pushing them forward as you exhale. Once you've built up some endurance in this exercise you can try using it in your stamina training. Whilst chain punching, assume the Golden Bridge stance and keep moving in this low position. Splicing a few minutes of this stance into your stamina work will markedly increase the staying power of your legs – not to mention shifting the workload up a gear.

Benefits

The tension created in the thighs and forearms speaks for itself. With early and continued practice, this simple and effective exercise will serve you well. You'll soon notice how the added power translates to easier kicking, climbing stairs and walking.

Power training 1.4 - Pushing Mountains
Level: Red

Explanation

Pushing Mountains is a Chi Kung exercise for building powerful arms. Its performance builds on the experience gained from practising the Prayer Press and the Golden Bridge. Using the principle of dynamic tension, resist your own movement as you attempt to push your palms away from you. If it helps, visualise actually pushing a really heavy object – like a mountain. The intensity, and therefore value, of this exercise is rounded off by assuming the Horse Stance, rather than the Character Two Stance. Now you've progressed through the Yellow level, use this stance whenever possible in your power training. When you practise the Prayer Press, assume the Horse Stance from this point onwards.

Performance

1. Open the Horse Stance.

2. Place your hands in front of your chest, palms outward and fingers pointing upward.

3. Inhale, breathing into your abdomen. Hold your breath for a moment and then begin to exhale.

4. Slowly, push your palms away from you, resisting the movement with your own strength.

5. When your arms are fully outstretched, pull your fingers back toward your body while pushing the heel of your palm forward a few times.

6. Resisting the movement, slowly clench your fingers into a fist and squeeze the fists as tight as possible a few times.

7. Inhale, breathing into your abdomen. Hold your breath for a moment and begin to exhale.

8. Once again resisting the movement with your own strength, pull your elbows backward until your hands return to your chest.

9. Unclench the fist and return the hands to the palm facing out position.

10. To begin with, pushing your arms out (and pulling them back), should take about two or three seconds. Clenching your fists should take about the same time. As you progress, slow the movement down and apply greater resistance.

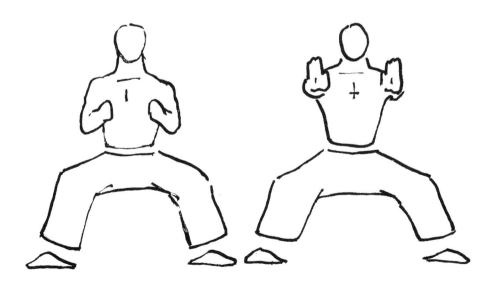

Variations

You can try alternately pushing out to the front, side, downward and upward, for well rounded conditioning of the upper body. You can also emphasise any part of the exercise which suits your training goals. Holding the open palm at arms length, pulling the fingers back and pushing the palm heel forward, is a great forearm exercise, as is forming the fist with dynamic tension. You could also throw in a few dynamic tension chain punches.

Benefits

Once you've mastered the dynamic tension concept, you can apply it to build strength and improve performance in any movement. Note the effect a few sessions of dynamic tension chain punching has on your stamina training. Not only will you be able to punch harder and longer, but dynamic tension will also develop added muscular control and physical awareness. The addition of the Horse Stance offers the opportunity to provide superb power conditioning to the entire body without ever lifting a weight.

Power training 1.5 - Abdominal curls
Level: Red

Explanation

Many martial arts place a premium on developing powerful muscles in the midsection. Much of the power for striking out with the hand or arm comes from the waist. Equally, a strong midsection supports the back and upper body stability, which allows you to take a punch if you have to. The major muscle group around the tummy is the Rectus Abdominis – or six-pack to the rest of us. These muscles draw together the rib cage and pelvis and help with the motion of sitting up. While very simple on the surface, the abdominal curl is extremely effective at concentrating your effort in the midsection.

Performance

1. Lie on the floor, placing your hands on your chest and drawing your feet up toward your buttocks.

2. Inhale, breathing into your abdomen. Hold your breath for a moment and begin to exhale.

3. Slowly lift your head, moving your chin to your chest. Then lift your upper back off the floor. You should only be able to move an inch or two.

4. Hold the final position for a second and then slowly lower yourself back to the starting position.

5. Lifting and lowering should take about 2 seconds each.

6. Start out with 5–7 repetitions, adding one a day until you can do 30 or more on the trot.

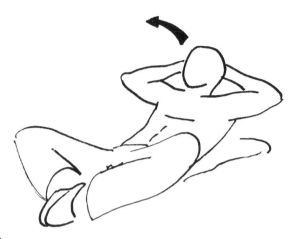

Variations

Like many of the exercises here, the abdominal curl lends itself to real growth. Once you've mastered the basics, you can add intensity to the curl by placing your hands on your shoulders and then stretching them out behind you. You can also move and hold the contracted position for extended periods. If you find this too easy, you can hold a heavy bag or weight on your chest. You can also try not to fully relax as you unfold to the starting position, instead maintain the tension on your rectus muscle and go straight into the next repetition. Equally, you can emphasise one side of your tummy by adding a slight twist at the top of the movement, pulling the right shoulder toward the left hip and so on.

Benefits

The midsection is the pivot around which the body turns. You'll soon find that regular and continued practice of this exercise will improve your performance in almost any activity. Your chances of back injury will fade dramatically, as will your waistline.

Power training 1.6 - The Empty Stance
Level: Red

Explanation

Once you've started to develop a solid foundation with the Horse Stance and Golden Bridge, the Empty Stance is the next evolution in training intensity. The Empty Stance develops power in the lower limbs to support the body during kicking. The Horse Stance spreads the body weight evenly over both legs. In the Empty Stance one leg carries the entire body weight and therefore receives more intense training. The supporting leg is said to be solid, because it carries the whole body weight. The other leg, which can be lifted from the ground without toppling over, is said to be empty. This exercise is complemented by the addition of the crane beak hand, not only adding upper body conditioning but also a touch of elegance to the whole movement.

Performance

1. Open the Horse Stance and hold this position for a few seconds.

2. Turn your head to the left and shift your body weight over onto your right leg.

3. Inhale into your abdomen. Hold your breath for a second and then slowly exhale.

4. As you shift your body weight, bring both hands up toward your chest, then two things happen at once:
   a. Push your left palm out over your left leg (just like Pushing Mountains exercise).

b. At the same time pinch the fingers of the right hand together to form a beak shape with the tips of the fingers pointing down. Now push the right hand back behind you turning the wrist anti-clockwise as you do, until the fingers are nearly pointing upward. You should feel tension in the right forearm and shoulder if you are doing this correctly.

5. Hold this final position for a count of 10 and return to the Horse Stance. Then repeat on the opposite side.

6. Start with 5 repetitions on each side. As you progress, work up to holding the Empty Stance for a minute or more. Also try to sink lower on the supporting, or solid leg.

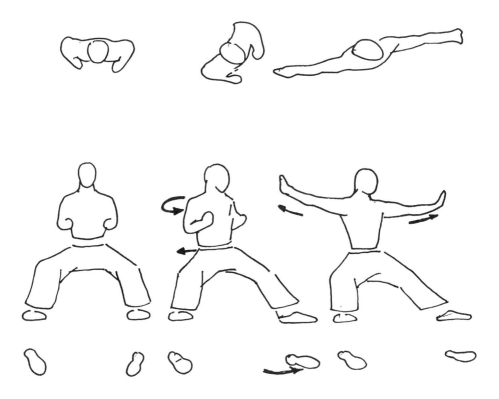

Variations

If you don't like the crane beak exercise just leave it out. It's not indispensable and can be replace with hands in the guard position. Once you've got the basic stance, you can try forcefully pointing the toes of the empty leg, like a ballet dancer. You can then try slightly lifting the empty leg off the floor and holding this position. This is a real challenge for both power and balance.

Benefits

All the benefits of Horse Stance training will be magnified by practising the Empty Stance. The added power, coordination and balance will also translate into enhanced performance during stamina exercises.

Power training 1.7 - Taming the Tiger
Level: Blue

Explanation

Because striking power is transmitted to an opponent through the arms, upper body strength is a key component of kung fu training. The development of upper body power through kung fu training is referred to as iron arm training. Taming the Tiger is central to iron arm training, and is similar to the regular press-up. Taming the Tiger has some subtle differences to the regular press-up, which not only make it a more productive exercise, but give it greater scope for growth.

Performance

1. Lie face down with your palms on the floor beside your chest and elbows pointing back towards your feet. Makes sure you are resting on the instep of the foot, not the toes as in regular press-ups (which makes them easier).

2. Inhale through your nose. Hold for a second then begin to exhale.

3. Slowly push your body off the floor, take a count of 5 to fully extend the arms.

4. Begin to lower your body at the same rate, but stop half way down and hold this position for a count of 5 before continuing to lower yourself to the floor.

5. Do not fully lower yourself to the floor, but hold yourself a few centimetres off the ground for a count of 5 before going straight into the next repetition.

6. Start out with 5–7 repetitions, gradually working up to 15–20. When you can perform 25 or more repetitions, try increasing the intensity of the exercise with some of the variations suggested below.

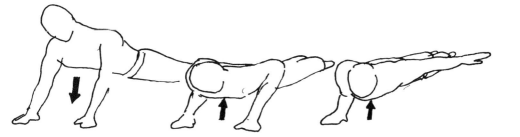

Variations

If you don't yet have the strength to fully 'tame the tiger', try performing the exercise leaning up against a wall. Gradually move your feet further back, so your body forms a greater angle with the wall as you become stronger. Soon you'll be taming the tiger with the best. If you are very strong, or want more challenge, try adding more stops as you lift and lower yourself. You can also perform the exercise with your feet elevated by placing them on a chair. This variation alters the leverage at the shoulder and places even greater emphasis on the arms. Alternatively, lean over on one arm so that is carries more weight, using the other for balance. Eventually, you can lift the balancing arm off the floor altogether. One-handed 'taming' is performed with the hand of the 'resting' arm held behind the head, touching the elbow on the floor at the end of the lowering phase. The final evolution is holding the resting arm straight out to your side and touching the floor with your palm at the bottom of the repetition.

Another interesting variation, which you can train on its own or slot into your stamina routine, is to try walking on your hands, from the low position of two-handed taming. Simply, hold your weight a few centimetres above the floor and then drag yourself along using your arms.

Benefits

Taming the Tiger will build tremendous power into your upper body. This will translate into other exercises, such as more powerful chain punches when stamina training, and the ease with which any daily activities involving carrying can be accomplished. The scope for growth in the exercise also ensures that it always provides a challenge. Once you can tame single-handed, you will truly have iron arms.

Power training 1.8 - Drawing the Moon
Level: Blue

Explanation

The major muscle of the tummy, the Rectus Abdominis, pulls the chest toward the pelvis. It also contracts statically, to support our posture when lifting the legs in kicking or when lying on the floor. Drawing the Moon is a deceptively simple exercise which takes advantage of this fact. Moving the legs to the side, during the upward and downward part of the movement also exercises the often neglected muscles at the side of the tummy.

Performance

1. Lie flat on your back, feet together, placing your hands on your tummy or by your sides.

2. Inhale through your nose. Hold for a second then begin to exhale.

3. Slowly lift your feet just off the floor and point your toes.

4. Moving in a clockwise direction describe a circle, or draw the moon, about two feet in diameter.

5. Each time you draw the moon should take no less than 10 seconds.

6. Start out with 5 repetitions clockwise and then anticlockwise.

7. Gradually increase the time it takes to draw the moon, working up to 30 seconds for each repetition.

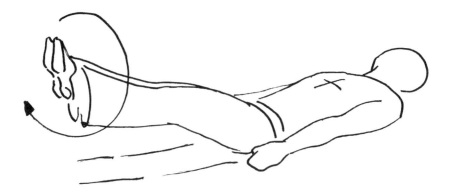

Variations

If you're not ready to draw the moon yet, try slowly lifting your feet straight up and down. Once you can perform 5 repetitions of 10 seconds each, 'draw' one moon before you rest. Then work up to more repetitions. As an alternative movement for the very strong, keep your feet at a constant height from the floor and move your legs over to one side and then the other. You could also try separating the feet and circling them in opposite directions at the same time (drawing two moons, as it were). A final evolution is to prop yourself up on your elbows while drawing the moon, placing even greater stress on the Rectus Abdominis.

Benefits

Drawing the Moon will build power and staying power into your waist. As the waist forms the vital link between the upper and lower body, this enhanced power will translate to better performance in almost any activity. The effect on your waistline will also be dramatic. Once you can draw the moon 10 times in each direction for 30 seconds you'll probably need to restock your wardrobe.

Power training 1.9 - The White Crane
Level: Blue

Explanation

Many movements and forms of kung fu are based on the observation of animals. White Crane borrows from the poise, powerful flapping motion of the wings and sudden strike of the beak. A fundamental training stance of White Crane is standing on one leg, as the bird itself can often be seen to do. The White Crane stance builds a strong foundation of strength and balance for posture and kicking. The entire body weight is carried on one leg. Bending the supporting knee places tremendous stress on the muscles of the thigh and buttock. Lifting the resting knee toward the chest emphasises the muscles of the thigh and waist.

Performance

1. Stand with your feet shoulder-width apart, arms by your sides.

2. Inhale through your nose. Hold for a second then begin to exhale.

3. Shift your weight onto your left foot and draw the right knee toward the chest while keeping your back straight.

4. Keeping your arms straight lift them out to the side (like a bird flapping its wings), keeping the fingers together and pointing at the ground.

5. Slightly bend the knee of the supporting leg until you feel tension in the thigh.

6. Start out holding this position for 30 seconds, then switch to the opposite leg and repeat.

7. Gradually increase the time you stand on each leg until you can do so for 3 minutes or more.

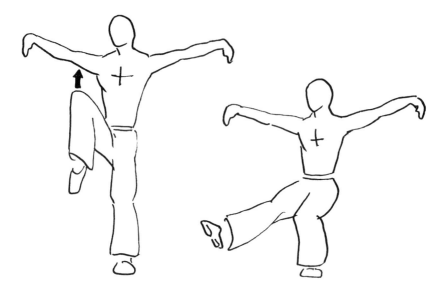

Variations

Once you can stand for 3 minutes, try slowly squatting as low as you can and returning to the starting position 5–10 times at the outset, then maintain the White Crane till the end of the 3 minutes. You can also try slowly extending the resting leg, as in kicking, a few times. In the fully evolved White Crane, keep the resting leg extended while you squat, so that it is parallel to the floor throughout.

Benefits

This is a tough exercise, but continued practice will deliver tremendous power, balance and poise. After time, most activities which emphasise the lower body will become effortless. Once mastered, you can use this stance while practising your upper body conditioning like the Prayer Press and Pushing Mountains.

Power training 1.10 - Muscle metamorphosis
Level: Black

Explanation

If you have progressed through the levels of power training you will have a full pallet of techniques at your disposal to develop your body. You should have also created a solid foundation of conditioning, enabling you to practise advanced techniques. Black level training introduces the concept of muscle metamorphosis. These techniques were among the first taught by Buddha to the monks of the Shaolin Temple. Muscle metamorphosis is several thousand years old and is the basis of all modern kung fu. Today these exercises offer advanced conditioning, drawing together the attributes of breathing, visualisation, stamina and power.

Performance

1. Place your feet together and close your eyes. Keep your mouth closed and touch the tip of your tongue to your pallet. Breathe slowly and deeply into your abdomen for 9 breaths. Clear your mind. Imagine a ball of powerful energy growing brighter in the base of your abdomen.

2. Keep your arms straight and raise them up in front of you so your hands are level with your shoulders. Form two fists with the thumb on top, and imagine your are holding a steel ball in each hand. Imagine the energy in your abdomen rushing through your chest and arms to your fists. Clench your fists as tight as you can, imagining yourself crushing the steel. Hold for a second and release. Keep your breathing slow and steady, only breathing out 70–80% before breathing in. Repeat up to 49 times before relaxing your arms to your sides.

3. Keep your arms at your sides and breathe steadily. Point your palms at the ground and your fingers straight forward. Once again, imagine energy rushing into your palms as you press the heel of the hand down and try to lift the fingertips forcefully. Repeat up to 49 times, then relax.

4. Smoothly open the Character Two Stance. Imagine the ball of energy sinking toward your thighs. Clench the pelvic floor muscles (the ones you clench when you're trying not to urinate), then the buttocks and then squeeze the knees together to tense the thighs as hard as you can. Hold for a few seconds, breathing steadily throughout, then relax in reverse order. 5–10 repeats will be more than enough.

5 Lift your arms out in front, so your hands are at mid-chest level, open with palms facing inward and elbows slightly bent. Imagine you're holding an invisible beach ball and you'll get the idea. Now, imagine energy rushing through your arms and flowing out of your finger tips. Then without actually moving your limbs clench your fists, arms and chest as if pushing against an immovable object as hard as you can. Hold for a few seconds, breathing steadily throughout, and relax before repeating 5–10 times.

6. Remain in this position opening the hands so the palms once again face inward. Sink your weight slightly by bending your knees. Breathe steadily and deeply, once again visualising energy rushing from your abdomen outward through all you limbs. Enjoy the tingling sensation in all your muscles as a result of this exercise. When you are ready, slowly lower your arms to your sides, stand upright and open your eyes.

7. As your condition improves, try to produce more powerful and longer periods of tension, working up to 5–15 seconds.

Variations

The muscle metamorphosis exercises can be practised in order, or in isolation. If you can't quite get the hang of clenching all the muscles of the chest and arms, try assuming the Prayer Press position and doing it that way until you're ready to practise the exercise as described.

Benefits

Muscle metamorphosis is extremely demanding. The strength for which Shaolin Monks are famous, is not gained easily. Metamorphosis exercise will, however, teach you to appreciate and coordinate breath, will and action as almost no other exercise can. You will reap the rewards in the enhanced performance of any activity – the pelvic floor exercise also has some very specific benefits you might notice with your partner! After a few weeks of consistent practice you'll notice the remarkable toning effect on your muscles. After a few months your sinews will have metamorphosed beyond recognition.

Special situations

We can always start again
Jack Korngold

Special situation 1.1 - Losing body fat

Explanation

The subject of weight control (more properly fat loss) has become a multi-billion dollar industry. The success of this industry is largely based on the desperation of its target audience coupled with an ignorance of the facts and unwillingness to put in the effort to achieve results. Despite an industry bent on convincing us of the existence of a magic formula, successful fat loss relies only on applying a few basic physical principles. Body fat is a mechanism we have evolved to store energy against less plentiful times in the future. When we are inactive or food is freely available, we tend to overeat and store fat. The plain truth is that fat loss is a simple and uncomplicated process. If you eat less and move more, you will lose fat.

Performance

1. Engage in vigorous stamina training for 30–40 minutes, 4–5 times each week. This burns energy and also signals a reduction in appetite.

2. Throw bursts of intense exercise into your stamina exercise. This helps burn energy faster and build muscle.

3. Exercise to build muscle. Muscle uses most of your energy at rest. More muscle burns more energy.

4. Stay active. This wastes extra energy and makes snacking and overeating less likely.

5. Build exercise into your schedule. Take the stairs instead of using the lift, etc.

6. Focus on foods with no added sugar and fat. Fruits, vegetables, whole grains and lean meat will hit the mark. These foods contain less energy and tend to be very filling. Fat and sugar also stimulate the appetite. Avoiding them will tend to mean eating less.

7. Avoid cakes, sweets, fried foods and fatty meat. These foods contain a great deal of energy for little volume. They stimulate the appetite and predispose you to overeating.

8. Avoid temptation. Keep only the foods you should eat in the house.

9. Eat regular, small meals. Remember, fat is a survival mechanism to protect you against starvation. Not eating puts your body on alert to famine. You will tend to overeat when you finally eat and feeling tired will mean you are less likely to exercise.

10. Don't try to lose weight quickly. This sends the message to your body that it is starving and should store fat whenever it gets the chance. Slowly ease the weight off and you are more likely to keep it off.

11. Eat what you want every now and again. Feeling deprived will only make you want to pig out.

12. Drink plenty of water. Dehydration will make you tired and can provoke a sensation of hunger.

13. Avoid fad diets, they will help you lose money rather than fat.

14. Learn about the physiology of body composition and exercise. The more you know, the more effective you can be.

Variations

There is an argument to reduce the amount of carbohydrate you eat and increase the level of protein. Essentially, excess carbohydrate signals a hormonal response, releasing insulin into the blood, which promotes fat storage. Insulin levels rise toward evening, so the idea is that you reduce the amounts of carbohydrate you eat as the day goes on. Checking food labels will quickly show you which foods contain the most carbohydrate. Protein requires a great deal of energy to break down and helps you to use up excess energy. Foods rich in protein are usually low in carbohydrate anyway, so changing the amount of one in your diet will normally affect the other.

Benefits

Carrying too much fat is associated with a range of serious illnesses. Even being slightly overweight can increase blood pressure, risk of heart disease and premature death. Carrying excess weight is tiring, reducing the energy you have for work or play. Being lean not only reduces the chance of illness, but increases energy and has a positive impact on your life as a whole.

Special situation 1.2 - Travel, jet lag and Deep Vein Thrombosis (DVT)

Explanation

The world is becoming an increasingly small place. Whether it's for business or leisure, we are travelling more than ever. With this new freedom comes a few problems. Travel often involves prolonged hours of enforced inactivity. If you fly long-haul you can find yourself sitting in one position for 8–12 hours. When you arrive it may be night-time but your body is used to eating breakfast. Even if you have the energy for exercise, there is no guarantee your destination will be furnished with a gym.

Performance

1. Whether sitting at the wheel of your car or on the red-eye to New York, you can use the sinew metamorphosis exercises to stretch and tone your muscles. You don't need much room and there is little movement involved.

2. On an airliner, you can move around so you can perform these exercises standing up. Tensing and relaxing the legs prevents pooling blood in the deep veins of the thigh and calf, reducing the risk of DVT.

3. In your car, you can supplement the sinew metamorphosis by straining against the wheel and pressing your legs against the sides of the foot well.

4. Remember that inactivity is a key ingredient in telling your body to gain fat. Be careful not to overeat at the same time. Avoiding in-flight alcohol and leaving the pudding out will help too.

5. Always seek an opportunity to practise, there is no reason you can't use this time to work on creating calm focus or practising abdominal breathing.

6. When you arrive on the far side of the world, the change in time zones may leave you feeling jaded and jet-lagged. This is simply the body's chemistry gearing up for sleep at it's usual time, regardless of the time where you are. East to west travel is typically the hardest for the air traveller because day breaks just when your body is expecting bedtime.

7. A session of stamina training can redress the worst of the feelings, as you start to adjust.

8. Also, avoid carbohydrate rich foods during the day, as these will promote changes in your body chemistry, leaving you feeling tired. Try and stay awake until your normal bedtime. Have a carbohydrate rich meal an hour or so before you retire and you should pass out nicely.

9. Of course, muscle metamorphosis allows you to maintain superb condition anywhere as it needs no special equipment. A few sessions while you are away, will fight off the worst travel has to offer.

Variations

You can apply these principles wherever you go in the world. The limitations of where you find yourself will dictate how you adapt your skills. If you have limited space, focus on those skills which require

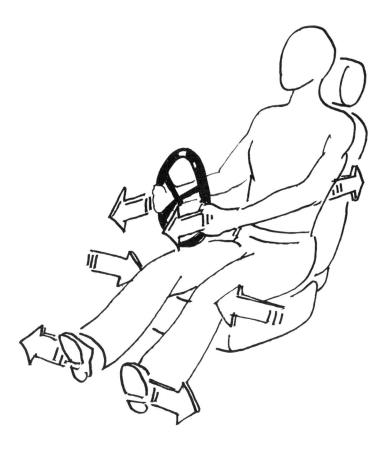

little movement: focus, breathing and sinew metamorphosis, until you have the freedom to express yourself with stamina training.

Benefits

Muscle metamorphosis allows you to maintain superb condition anywhere, anytime.

Special situation 1.3 - In a hurry

Explanation

There never seems to be enough time. There is always one more thing to do. The pace of life for most of us has increased tremendously. In response to an increasingly global economy, and rising expectations, we are all being driven to become busier. This often leads to some activities being sacrificed. These may well be the very activities we enjoy or those that benefit us the most. Modern life, and especially the twenty-first century workplace, predisposes us to inactivity and stress. At the same time our physical condition is suffering. No matter how busy you get, scheduling exercise into your routine offers real benefits to your energy levels, health and focus.

Performance

1. A workout is a workout. Even if you can only afford 15–10 minutes stamina and 5 minutes strength training – it all helps.

2. Exercise is exercise. You can work it into your daily activities. Take the stairs instead of the lift. Walk or cycle rather than taking the car.

3. There will always be something else you could be doing but schedule exercise into your diary even if the sessions are short. Keep a regular routine and make it a priority – soon it will become a habit.

4. If time pressure means you can't get through a full routine, split it up. Focus on your lower body in one session, emphasising kicks and lower limb strength exercises, and on your upper body in the next session.

5. The results of exercise are dose related. Benefits come from how hard, often and long you train. To some extent these are interchangeable. Train harder and more frequently when you have more time. Weekends and days off are excellent times to squeeze in a few training sessions. Keep things ticking over with lighter work when you are busy.

Variations

Your own schedule will dictate how you adapt your own exercise routine. So long as you follow the basic principles, there are no firm rules. Experience will soon tell you how much exercise you need to reach your goals, or how little you require to maintain them when you arrive.

Benefits

Having mastered the principles of muscle metamorphosis, you can adapt them to the particular pressures of your own lifestyle. Rather than a rigid prescription for exercise, you can develop your own unique strategy.

Special situation 1.4 - Lifetime good health

Explanation

From the moment of conception, the human body is subject to a remarkable process of growth, development and ageing. No aspect of our physiology or psychology is exempt from these effects. It follows that we may respond differently to the demands of daily life depending upon our age, gender and circumstances. Equally, our preparedness to meet the challenges of life tomorrow may well depend on the efforts we make today.

Performance

1. Values promoted by our parents and role models will usually form the basis for those displayed by children as they grow-up. If these tendencies lead to poor physical development and obesity, they can establish a self-reinforcing cycle which is very hard to break in adulthood. Parents and adult role models have a golden opportunity to help children get a head start on a lifetime of good health. Childhood defines the patterns carried into adult life.

2. Children are usually not interested in the reasons to avoid sweets and fatty foods: the bottom line is they taste good. Equally, exercise is hard work and bites into playtime. The key to establishing good habits early on is a role model emphasizing moderate indulgence and fun in movement. Having played the video game, why not challenge a recreation of the *SmackDown* in real life? This also has the effect of getting the adult children off the sofa. Carry the same principles over into the mealtimes – Bruce Lee did not get his washboard abs from eating candy bars – and you've got a plan that's coming together.

3. The transition to adolescence heralds a greater distinction between genders. Exercise during this period can be a useful way to understand these changes, build confidence and release some of the tension from raging hormones. Importantly, the transition to adulthood probably suggests a different emphasis in exercise for men and women. Given the greater risk of heart disease faced simply by being male, men should be sure to include some regular aerobic exercise in their routine. The loss of bone mass and lean tissue associated with aging in women may well be offset by early and continued emphasis on power training. The foundations for health in later life, as well as the patterns of behaviour to maintain them, are reinforced here.

4. Not content with promoting bone and muscle loss in old age, nature also deals the female of the species a trial by childbirth. Pregnancy does not, and should not, preclude physical exercise at all. Almost any kind of exercise is completely safe up until a few weeks before birth. Exercise helps mothers adjust to the physical challenges of pregnancy, may make labour easier to endure, and should stimulate faster recovery.

5. Weakness and infirmity are not the inevitable conclusions of old age, but usually the consequences of choices made while younger. While there may be some obligatory loss of physical capacity with age, this can be delayed or avoided with regular exercise and a healthy lifestyle. Over 60 is not over the hill and retirement offers a fantastic opportunity to be physical. Muscle, joint and bone health seem to suffer more with age than heart and lung function, so an emphasis on building strength and mobility seems very much in order for more senior participants.

Variations

In addition to a shifting emphasis on exercise across our lifetime, it does appear there are a few other lifestyle factors strongly associated with robust good health at any age. In no particular order these are: eat regular meals and don't skip breakfast, drink plenty of water, don't smoke, drink alcohol in moderation, take regular exercise, keep regular sleeping patterns and aim for eight hours a night, maintain a positive outlook on life. Many of these factors are almost self-evident, but it doesn't hurt to remind ourselves.

Benefits

Vigorous good health is among the greatest assets you can possess. Any amount of wealth becomes meaningless when you cannot exploit it. Even the closest relationships suffer when you cannot fully engage in them. Whatever your aspirations, at any age, you will be handsomely rewarded by attaining a higher level of physical and mental readiness.

Wing Chun books

***Beginning Wing Chun: Why Wing Chun Works* by Alan Gibson.** The most comprehensive Wing Chun book available... A functional reference that gets to the heart of Wing Chun.

***Simple Thinking, Intelligent Fighters* by Alan Gibson.** Clear guidelines on how to develop the techniques and concepts shown in the first book. Easy to read and absorb.

***The Wing Chun Forms: Combat Textbooks* by Alan Gibson.** A detailed journey through the first two forms and the Wooden Dummy, using practical applications.

Wing Chun DVDs

***Wing Chun – In a Class of its Own* by Alan Gibson.** An overview of the Wing Chun system; Siu Nim Tao and Cham Kiu demonstrated. All the major drills and theories are investigated.

***Wing Chun – Keeping It Real!* by Alan Gibson.** Featuring the wooden dummy form and application. Also pressure testing drills.

***Improving Wing Chun Forms* by Alan Gibson.** All six Wing Chun forms demonstrated clearly from start to finish. Commentary on each form.

***Improving Wing Chun Drills* by Alan Gibson.** All the major Wing Chun drills. Clearly filmed and explained from multiple angles to facilitate easy learning.

***Improving Wing Chun Chi Sau* by Alan Gibson.** How to train and improve your fighting skill through Chi Sau. Includes many drills and common mistakes.

Cross Training in Martial Arts **by Jamie Clubb, Geoff Thompson, Peter Consterdine, Rick Young, Alan Gibson, Iain Abernethy, Shihan Chris Rowen, Mo Teague.** Including never seen before interviews, techniques and more!

The Master's Seminar **by Alan Gibson.** Wing Chun key footwork concepts that can help anyone improve their art.

Beginning Wing Chun **by Alan Gibson.** A syllabus-based training film showing the progression of practice and understanding of Wing Chun.

Posters

Siu Nim Tao and Cham Kiu. Top quality, large (A1) size posters of the forms.

Web

All merchandise is available to order from The Wing Chun Federation website: **www.wingchun.org.uk**

Notes

Notes

Notes

Visit us at
mindandbodymetamorphosis.co.uk
or
drmatthewmills.co.uk